Praise for

When Faith Faces Cancer

"Join Valerie on her cancer journey and walk with her through the amazing story of God's faithfulness to her in the phases of diagnosis, surgery, chemotherapy and reconstruction. Along the way there is an intimate sharing of her personal struggles, and powerful testimonies of the Lord's faithfulness, intertwined with many deep reflections and meditations on the truths of Scripture. I have known Valerie since she joined us in Turkey in the early 1990's and heartily recommend this book as a resource for anyone struggling with life's challenges."

Julyan Lidstone, author, speaker, and leader in Operation Mobilization International

"As a cancer survivor myself, I identified with the struggles Valerie describes. I nodded at her recounting of the emotional ups and downs that surround the experience of a cancer diagnosis and treatment. Valerie gives us an inside view of what it fells like to wrestle with cancer while experiencing faith in Christ as our companion. The stories from others bring further encouragement and hope for us as we encounter the challenging circumstances of life. I recommend that you read this book."

Bill Smith, Director, The C.S. Lewis Institute Atlanta

© 2025 by Valerie Huff
All rights reserved. No part of this publication may be reproduced, stored in a retrieval system, or transmitted in any form-electronic, mechanical, photocopying, recording, or otherwise-without the prior written permission of the author, except for brief quotations in reviews or articles.

Unless otherwise indicated, all scripture quotations are from the Holy Bible, New International Version®, NIV®
©1973, 1978, 1984, 2011 by Biblica, Inc.™

Scripture quotes marked NASB are from the New American Standard Bible®
©1960, 1962, 1963, 1968, 1971, 1972, 1973, 1975, 1977, 1995, 2020 by the Lockman Foundation. All rights reserved.

ISBN: 9798296838445

When Faith Faces Cancer

==================

Scriptures and Stories that Inspire Transformation

Valerie Huff

Acknowledgements

A heartfelt thanks go to my family that surrounded me through the cancer journey.
To my husband, who was there for me from the beginning, a calm presence with words of hope and encouragement.
To family, friends, neighbors, and my tennis team who showered me with food, gifts, cards, and texts.
To my mother and father, for their constant love and prayers.

Thanks to Angela Olson Brown and Karen Dial who helped with initial edits of this book.
To my daughters Abigail and Arianna Huff who provided their beautiful illustrations.
To my dear friends who provided their inspiring stories included in this book.
To Julyan and Bill for their endorsements.
To Angela Kleman, for the final editing.

Contents

Preface / 1
Introduction / 3
Chapter 1   In His Hand / 5
Chapter 2   God Is a Loving Father / 7
Chapter 3   The Bride and Groom / 11
Chapter 4   He Spreads His Wings / 15
Chapter 5   The Vintner and Vineyard / 19
Chapter 6   The Vine and Branches / 23
Chapter 7   The Potter and Clay / 27
Chapter 8   The Good Shepherd and Sheep / 31
Chapter 9   Trust and Surrender / 35
Chapter 10 Anxiety / 41
Chapter 11 Disease or Dis-ease? / 47
Chapter 12 Distractions / 51
Chapter 13 Soul Healing Under the Great Surgeon's Knife / 57
Chapter 14 Turkish Carpets, Canvases, and Suffering / 65
Chapter 15 The Powerful Effect of Thanksgiving / 69
Chapter 16 Contentment / 77
Chapter 17 Teatime with God / 79
Chapter 18 Joy in the Midst of Weakness / 83
Chapter 19 Cancer… a Platform to Help Others / 89
Chapter 20 Others' Stories / 93
Chapter 21 When Cancer Ends in Death / 115
Chapter 22 Practical Tips / 119
Closing   / 123
Citations   / 125

Preface

As you walk with the One who stated, "I am the Way, the Truth, and the Life," I pray that God will use your cancer journey as a transformative exploration, leading you to experience the life and fullness of Jesus himself. I found this Abundant Life who is Christ years ago. Since then, I have continually found him faithful to help me grow in a deeper understanding of what it means to walk with him.

While single in my twenties and early thirties, I lived in other countries and cultures and used this opportunity to share this gift of abundant life with others. God used that period of life to profoundly shape my worldview and heart for the nations, influencing much of my lifestyle today. Now in my late fifties, I have a full and busy life as a homemaker, wife, mom of three, and part-time Registered Dietitian. Besides keeping up with family and work, I enjoy volunteering in my community.

In 2022, I was diagnosed with breast cancer. Although the initial shock and subsequent surgeries and treatments were filled with challenges and struggles, I am grateful for all the work God poured into me, leading me to greater joy. Looking back over the decades, I see how God has been faithful in using crises to help me experience more of him. Walking though breast cancer was no different.

My story is interwoven with various threads of insights which God has taught me along the way. You'll find stories and metaphors from my oversees experience, scripture readings, questions for reflection, as well as journaling spaces to assist you in your own unique journey.

No matter where you are in your spiritual quest, rest assured that God is directing your story and seeking to push you toward the higher plane of abundant life. To begin, simply place your hand in his.

When Faith Faces Cancer

Introduction
Abundant Life

Jesus makes a repeated and remarkable promise throughout the New Testament. He promises life to all who believe in him, but this is no ordinary life. As we see throughout the New Testament, three Greek words are used to convey the idea of life. One is *bios*, which refers to the idea of biological life.[1] Another is *psuche (or psyche)*, which refers to the idea of a soul, or that which makes up the mind, emotion, and will of a person.[2] Then we see the word *zoe*. Standing above and beyond the other two, *zoe* refers to the life of God, uncreated, full, supreme, and transcendently divine. This is the word Jesus uses constantly to describe life in himself and the quality of life he longs to impart to us. *Zoe comes from and is sustained by God's self-existent life.*[3] God used my cancer journey to help me grow in his abundant life.

In *Mere Christianity*, one of my favorite authors, C.S. Lewis, compares *bios* and *zoe* in this way:

The spiritual life which is in God from all eternity, and which made the whole natural universe is *zoe*. Bios has, to be sure, a certain shadowy or symbolic resemblance to Zoe; but only the sort of resemblance there is between a photo and a place, or a statue and a man. A man who changed from having bios to having Zoe would have gone through as big a change as a statue which changed from being a carved stone to being a real man.[4]

Zoe is the higher plane of dimensional life that Christ promises to those who believe in him. He states, "The thief comes only to steal, kill, and destroy; I come so that they would have life (zoe), and have it abundantly" (John 10:10, NASB).

Not only does Jesus want to impart this divine quality of zoe life to us but also wants to give it *abundantly*. The word *abundantly*, which is the Greek *perissos* in the New Testament, can be translated, "all around, excess, more than, beyond what is anticipated, or exceeding expectation."[5] We can imagine the impact of Jesus' words to the original audience, which may have sounded something like, "I have come so that those who believe in me will continuously have my overflowing, divine life within themselves that exceeds their expectations." One of the wonderful things about this gift of abundant life is it is dependent on God's life and not our physical condition or health. Even in the midst of cancer one may experience zoe.

Chapter 1
In His Hand

My cancer journey began in the summer of 2022 in Costa Rica. My husband and I, with our two teenage girls, vacationed there while our oldest teenager, our son, was away at Georgia's Governor's Honors Program. On one of our Costa Rican adventures, we ziplined across valleys, from mountain to mountain, on cables almost a half-mile long! Just before we flung ourselves across the immense expanses, we were photographed in a statue of an enormous weather-beaten concrete hand.

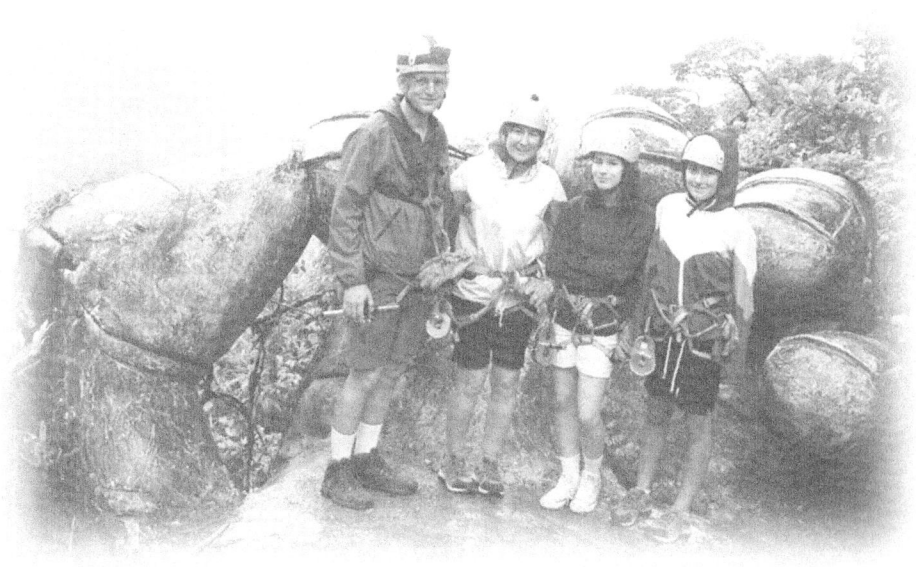

The hand—known as "La Mano Del Arenal" or "The Owner of the Mount,"—provided a perfect photoshoot for our family as we hopped into the hand, we relished the opportunity to be photographed in this unique place and time. The sight of the giant concrete hand reaching up through the dense green vegetation with a view of the vast valley in the background was truly a sight to behold. As we stood there in the palm of that great hand, I had three thoughts that hit me all at once:

> A trial will come soon which will affect our whole family.
> Jesus is with us.
> We are in his hand.

The thoughts dissipated as quickly as they'd formed, like the misty clouds covering the skies above, leaving me with complete peace and confidence. Little did I know of the storm that would envelop our lives just six weeks later.

Chapter 2
God Is a Loving Father ... and Other Relationship Analogies

A constant theme runs through the Bible, full of life and purpose, communicating the grand design of God for us. This theme is God's redemption, that is, his radical love for his creation, and how he pursues us by ransoming us at the price of his own life. God illustrates his care and love for us in the rich imagery and relationships we see throughout his word. Through these relationship analogies and metaphors, we discern the ways God works in our individual lives. Each type reveals a unique facet of the multisided diamond that our abundant life in Christ is like. These metaphors and analogies have been significant to me over the years and especially during my cancer journey.

The father/child relationship analogy is one of the most prevalent which God weaves throughout the Old and New Testaments. As a good father has compassion on his children, so God has compassion on us. God is eager to adopt us into his family through new life in his Son, Jesus Christ. God is the perfect Father, whose love surpasses the love of the very best earthly father or any human relationship. Psalm 103:13 promises, "Just as a father has compassion on his children, so the Lord has compassion on those who fear him." Little did I know I'd soon hold fast to this promise, as the darkest days of my cancer journey were just around the corner. This truth of him as a compassionate father, who not only cares, but is in control of the details of my life, was a stabilizing reality releasing me from the choke hold of worry and anxiety.

When the news of the diagnosis shook me to the core and literally knocked the breath out of me, the foundation of his sovereignty, fatherhood, and compassion stood fast. After receiving the dreadful diagnosis, I found I was unable to shake the constant barrage of anxious thoughts and the downward spiral of worry. This became evident after reading the biopsy report a few days later: "invasive carcinoma" with "rapidly dividing mitotic structures." Again, I felt my head swirl around with this uncertain news. This new reality I was living in caused me to continually turn to my loving Heavenly Father as my foundation and rock in the sea of chaos. Each time I felt overwhelmed I turned to him and immersed myself in his word and the truth of his sovereign love. Time with God in his word proved to be transformative to my mind and heart, enabling me to surrender my fears to him and receive his peace.

~Reflect~

Because you are his sons, God sent the Spirit of his Son into our hearts, the Spirit who calls out, "Abba, Father." (Galatians 4:6)

[14] For those who are led by the Spirit of God are the children of God. [15] The Spirit you received does not make you slaves, so that you live in fear again; rather, the Spirit you received brought about your adoption to sonship. And by him we cry, "Abba, Father." [16] The Spirit himself testifies with our spirit that we are God's children. [17] Now if we are children, then we are heirs—heirs of God and co-heirs with Christ, if indeed we share in his sufferings in order that we may also share in his glory. (Romans 8:14-17)

[12] Yet to all who did receive him, to those who believed in his name, he gave the right to become children of God— [13] children born not of natural descent, nor of human decision or a husband's will, but born of God. (John 1:12,13)

As a father has compassion on his children, so the Lord has compassion on those who fear him... .(Psalm 103:13)

See what great love the Father has lavished on us, that we should be called children of God! And that is what we are! The reason the world does not know us is that it did not know him. (1 John 3:1)

With the previous verses in mind, list the characteristics of a child of God.

What are the promises for the child of God?

What characteristics and actions of the Father do we see in these Scriptures?

What aspects of God's father heart towards us is most meaningful to you and why?

When Faith Faces Cancer

Chapter 3
The Bride and Groom

As a groom rejoices over his bride and is committed in covenant relationship to her, God seeks a similar covenant with a pure and devoted spiritual bride, that is, his body of believers, made up of individuals who are joined in oneness with him. "... as a bridegroom rejoices over his bride, so will your God rejoice over you" (Isaiah 62:5).

It's an amazing truth that God rejoices over us. He not only loves us but likes and delights in us! He pursues us to draw us into a covenant relationship with himself. Do you know that God is happy just to be with you? The delightfulness of my relationship with Jesus, my bridegroom, brought unusual peace in the midst of medical visits, tests, surgeries, and so many other challenges that come with cancer.

The first time I knew of the very real possibility that I could have breast cancer was at a diagnostic mammogram appointment. The doctor spoke of "suspicious calcifications" and with a deeply concerned look in her eyes, added "I will give it a fifty-fifty chance it's cancer." Instantly, I knew what she was really trying to say was, "I think it's probably cancer; we'll need to confirm with a biopsy."

At the biopsy appointment the next day, a sense of dread penetrated me. As they took my blood pressure at the beginning, I was shocked that it was so high. Normally, my blood pressure sits around the low side of normal. "That can't be right," I insisted. "Can you do that over?" My request only brought on a slightly higher reading! No matter how many deep breaths or scenes of a beautiful Caribbean beach I imagined, I couldn't bring it down. With a sense of desperation I prayed,

"Lord Jesus, you are my future bridegroom,
I'm one with you and I throw myself upon your arms of grace.
No matter what happens I am with you,
and you are in control over all things."

I prayed this prayer with the image of his mighty arms underneath me as I climbed upon the elevated table on all fours. The nurse told me to lie down on my tummy, face down in a very uncomfortable position, and not to move for an extended period of time. The initial breast biopsy was proving to be a more difficult experience than I had imagined, and I had not even felt the piercing jab of the needle yet!

The image and knowledge of Jesus as my bridegroom and my future glory with him, and that he is touched by every form of suffering we experience brought a deep peace that he was with me, and this was all from him. God used the soft, kind voice of one of the nurses to remind me that Jesus is gentle and merciful with those who suffer, and he understands the trials we walk through. A scripture I had memorized years ago came to my mind:

> "Take my yoke upon you and learn from me,
> for I am gentle and humble in heart,
> and you will find rest for your souls" (Jesus in Matthew 11:29).

Experiencing God and his presence knows no bounds as we immerse ourselves in his word and promises. No matter where we go or what we experience in the cancer trial, we always have access to his presence as we pray, connect with him, and read his word. If we are united with Christ, we encounter a deeper spiritual bond than any marriage we can experience on this earth. Our oneness with him goes deeper and transforms every area of our life, as his covenant relationship with us is unchanging.

We look forward to the marriage supper of the Lamb (called *the Lamb* because he was the sacrifice for our sins), as Revelation 19:7 points us to this future hope: "Let us rejoice and be glad, for the marriage of the Lamb has come, and his bride (his body, the church) has made herself ready."

~Reflect~

As a young man marries a young woman,
  so will your Builder marry you;

Scriptures and Stories That Inspire Transformation

as a bridegroom rejoices over his bride,
   so will your God rejoice over you. (Isaiah 62:5)

I delight greatly in the Lord;
   my soul rejoices in my God.
For he has clothed me with garments of salvation
   and arrayed me in a robe of his righteousness,
as a bridegroom adorns his head like a priest,
   and as a bride adorns herself with her jewels. (Isaiah 61:10)

I am jealous for you with a godly jealousy. I promised you to one husband, to Christ, so that I might present you as a pure virgin to him. But I am afraid that just as Eve was deceived by the serpent's cunning, your minds may somehow be led astray from your sincere and pure devotion to Christ. For if someone comes to you and preaches a Jesus other than the Jesus we preached, or if you receive a different spirit from the Spirit you received, or a different gospel from the one you accepted, you put up with it easily enough. (2 Corinthians 11:2-4)

But whoever is united with the Lord is one with him in spirit. (1 Corinthians 6:17)

Husbands, love your wives, just as Christ loved the church and gave himself up for her to make her holy, cleansing her by the washing with water through the word, and to present her to himself as a radiant church, without stain or wrinkle or any other blemish, but holy and blameless. In this same way, husbands ought to love their wives as their own bodies. He who loves his wife loves himself. (Ephesian 5:25-28)

Then I heard what sounded like a great multitude, like the roar of rushing waters and like loud peals of thunder, shouting:
Hallelujah!
   For our Lord God Almighty reigns.
Let us rejoice and be glad
   and give him glory!

For the wedding of the Lamb has come,
    and his bride has made herself ready.
Fine linen, bright and clean,
    was given her to wear. (Revelation 19:7)

With the previous verses in mind, describe the actions and attitudes of God toward his own.

How are these like an earthly bridegroom with his bride?

What actions and responsibilities of the bride do we see in the verses above?

Chapter 4
He Spreads His Wings

    A mother hen spreads her wings over her chicks to protect them from the elements and an eagle flies under her young to lift them up in the air as they learn to fly. These analogies beautifully illustrate how God protects his own. The relationship analogy of God spreading his wings over us is seen many times in the Old Testament and used by Jesus when he wept over Jerusalem (Matthew 23:37). Jesus stated at that time, "… how often I have longed to gather your children together as a hen gathers her chicks under her wings… ." In the same way, God longs to gather each of us under his wings through salvation which is found in Christ.

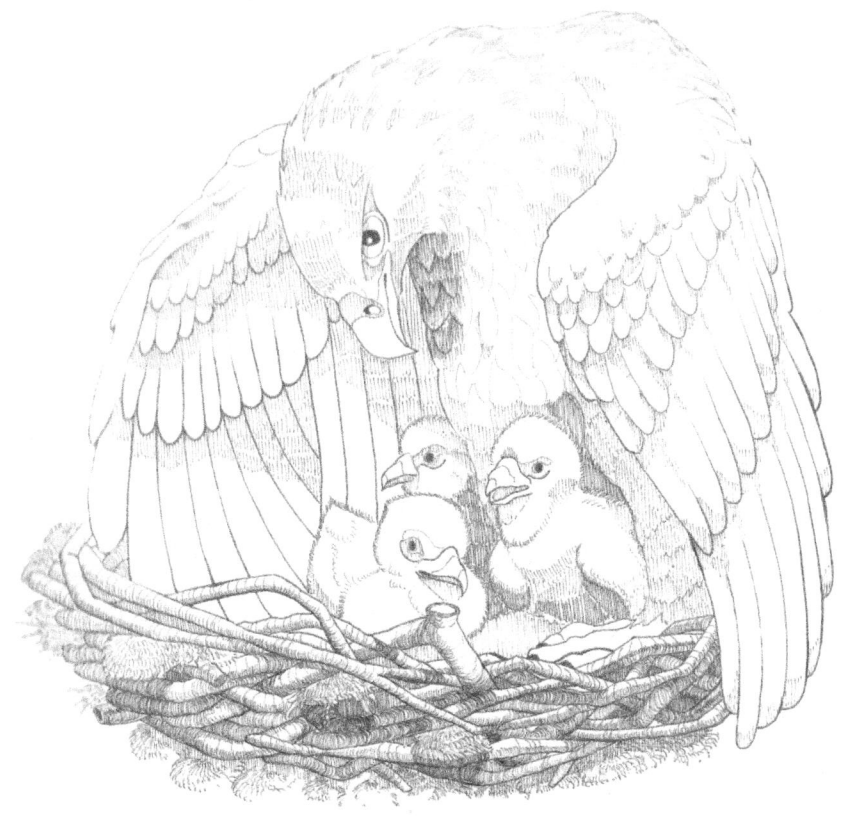

I imagined myself taking refuge under his wings many times during the cancer journey when fear threatened to enfold me. Several nights during my chemo treatments, I woke up with mild tremors, possibly exhibiting symptoms of a Taxol reaction, which the nurses warned me about. Facing this fear and the possibility of an ER visit, I prayed, thanking God that he is my deliverer and asking him to calm these reactions. Each time, the shaking subsided. The image of his wings spread over me like a blanket and filled my mind as I drifted back into a peaceful sleep.

~Reflect~

Keep me as the apple of your eye; hide me in the shadow of your wings. You are my hiding place; you will protect me from trouble and surround me with songs of deliverance. (Psalm 17:8)

How priceless is your unfailing love, O God! People take refuge in the shadow of your wings. (Psalm 32:7)

Have mercy on me, my God, have mercy on me, for in you I take refuge. I will take refuge in the shadow of your wings until the disaster has passed. (Psalm 57:1)

I long to dwell in your tent forever and take refuge in the shelter of your wings. (Psalm 61:4)

Because you are my help, I sing in the shadow of your wings. (Psalm 63:7)

He will cover you with his feathers, and under his wings you will find refuge, his faithfulness will be your shield and rampart. (Psalm 91:4)

Like an eagle that stirs up its nest and hovers over its young, that spreads its wings to catch them and carries them aloft .... (Deuteronomy 32:11)

Write the insights you see in the way God cares for us based on the previous verses.

List a few of God's attributes and characteristics you see in the previous verses.

Write out a prayer of thanksgiving based on these facts.

When Faith Faces Cancer

Chapter 5
The Vintner and Vineyard

A vintner works hard to dig up and clear stones in a field he's chosen for his vineyard. When the soil is ready, he plants his vines in the fertile ground, watches over them, and tends them carefully to produce grapes. Similarly, God carefully works to prepare the best environment within our heart to produce fruit. Galatians 5:22-24 describes this life-giving fruit as love, joy, peace, patience, kindness, goodness, faithfulness, gentleness, and self-control. If we know Christ personally, the Holy Spirit causes these fruitful characteristics to develop and grow in us, transforming us to be more like Jesus each day. Other fruit includes our godly influence upon others and all those who come to believe and follow Christ through our stories.

The vintner/vineyard imagery emphasizes the hard work of farming and preparing the soil through tilling and removing stones and obstacles out of the way. This enables the Master Grower to do his work to produce fruit in a prepared heart. In the Old Testament, Isaiah 5:1-4 uses this analogy about the vineyard: "He dug it up, cleared it of stones, and planted it with the choicest vines. He built a watchtower in it and cut out a winepress as well. Then he looked for a crop of good grapes … ."

In our hearts, we might struggle with bitterness toward God and others, unbelief about God's goodness to us, apathy about his priorities and plans, lack of love towards others, and idols of wealth and comfort that we put ahead of following and obeying Christ. All are examples of stones and rocks that he will remove from the soil of our heart—if we let him—to make it fertile for the growth of the fruit of his Spirit. The Lord helped me to see stones and rocks of self-absorption, pride, and apathy in the soil of my heart along the path of my cancer journey.

These stones and rocks were preventing his deeper work of growth in my life. I knew through this process of digging, clearing, and pruning, God was working to get rid of my obstacles. Granted, the digging, clearing, and pruning can be painful, but the results that God desires are worth it. Jesus uses this analogy in his parable in Luke 8:4-15 about the four types of soils.

~Reflect~

[4] While a large crowd was gathering and people were coming to Jesus from town after town, he told this parable: [5] "A farmer went out to sow his seed. As he was scattering the seed, some fell along the path; it was trampled on, and the birds ate it up. [6] Some fell on rocky ground, and when it came up, the plants withered because they had no moisture. [7] Other seed fell among thorns, which grew up with it and choked the plants. [8] Still other seed fell on good soil. It came up and yielded a crop, a hundred times more than was sown"
When he said this, he called out, "Whoever has ears to hear, let them hear."
[9] His disciples asked him what this parable meant. [10] He said, "The knowledge of the secrets of the kingdom of God has been given to you, but to others I speak in parables, so that,
"'though seeing, they may not see;
   though hearing, they may not understand.'
[11] "This is the meaning of the parable: The seed is the word of God.
[12] Those along the path are the ones who hear, and then the devil comes and takes away the word from their hearts, so that they may not believe and be saved. [13] Those on the rocky ground are the ones who receive the word with joy when they hear it, but they have no root. They believe for a while, but in the time of testing they fall away. [14] The seed that fell among thorns stands for those who hear, but as they go on their way they are choked by life's worries, riches and pleasures, and they do not mature. [15] But the seed on good soil stands for those with a noble and good heart, who hear the word, retain it, and by persevering produce a crop." (Luke 8:4-15)

List the four types of soils and the explanation Jesus gives for each.

List the obstacles in the first three soils that keep them from bearing fruit.

Describe the heart and behavior of the one who produces fruit, which is seen in the fourth type of soil.

Reflect on each type of soil and ask God to show you what obstacles and hindrances keep you from bearing fruit. List them here and ask God to transform each one.

Chapter 6
The Vine and Branches

As the grapevine supplies the branches with all the nourishment it needs, and the branch is completely dependent on the vine for its life, so are we dependent upon Christ, receiving life from him. This is where Jesus presents the idea of abiding in him. "Abide in Me, and I in you. As the branch cannot bear fruit of itself, unless it abides in the vine, neither can you, unless you abide in Me…apart from Me you can do nothing" (John. 15:4,5 NASB).

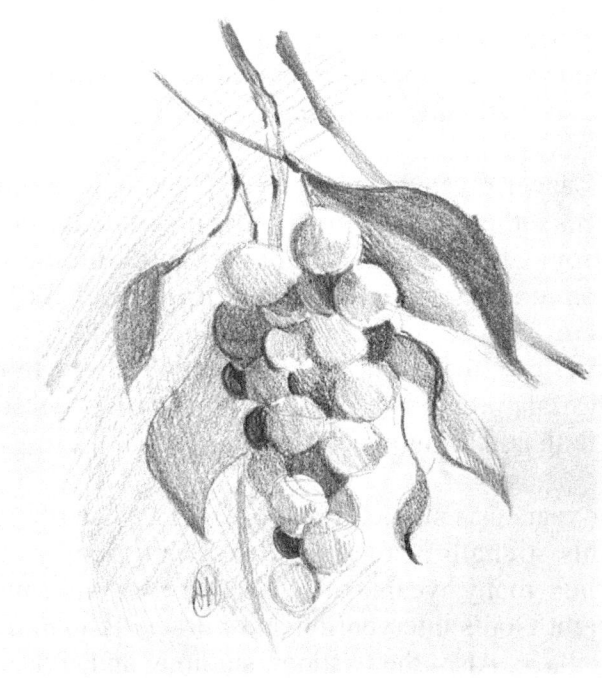

The analogy of the vine and the branches begs the question, "Am I in Christ?" We see in this Scripture Jesus' explanation that our own goodness and righteousness are insufficient for God's standards. We have all sinned, and our hearts are unable to produce the kind of goodness and righteousness that God requires. Romans 8:6 explains: "The mind (or heart) governed by the flesh is death, but the mind governed by the Spirit is life and peace. The mind governed by the flesh is hostile to God; it does not submit to God's law, nor can it do so."

Jesus is referring to the new life in himself and the fruit that is produced when his Spirit takes residence in the soul of a person through the "washing of rebirth and renewal by the Holy Spirit" (Titus 3:5). Jesus further speaks of this new life when he says to Nicodemus in John 3:3: "Very truly I tell you, no one can see the Kingdom of God unless they are born again."

Abiding in Christ is maintained when we rely on Christ's power through his Spirit in us as we walk with him in faith. As we spend time with him in Bible reading and prayer, depending on him for our needs, we receive his source of grace, strength, love, and peace.

Going through cancer revealed areas where I had unknowingly looked to my own resources rather than to Christ. These included a tendency toward independence from God and neglecting his counsel through prayer. These are two very common inclinations of the human heart for all of us. God graciously used my cancer to make me experience that he is my source and my own resources eventually ran dry. I noticed the same thing when God led me through trials previously in my life. They always serve to purify and renew my faith and bring me closer to himself.

In my earlier years as a single, living overseas, I had often felt the need to draw from his strength in the midst of feeling lonely and homesick. Similarly, during many years of childlessness, my husband and I continually sought God's intervention and miracle to give us the children he wanted us to have. Also, the wisdom, stamina, and consistency needed for motherhood, especially when our kids were young, brought me to my knees in prayer often. Education decisions for our kids led me into his presence often, seeking his wisdom and direction for the right path. All these challenges served to make me feel keenly my need to abide in Christ and receive from him.

God uses all things in our lives—every challenge and source of stress—to help us depend more on him if our hearts are humble enough to yield to the process. I knew very soon in the cancer journey that the resources needed to live with emotional margin, love my family well, accept the future with open hands, and even to flourish emotionally and spiritually had to come from God's supply of strength and not my own.

~Reflect~

But the fruit of the Spirit is love, joy, peace, patience, kindness, goodness, faithfulness, gentleness, and self-control.... (Galatians 5:22)

But blessed is the one who trusts in the Lord, whose confidence is in him. They will be like a tree planted by the water that sends out its roots by the stream. It does not fear when heat comes; its leaves are always green. It has no worries in a year of drought and never fails to bear fruit. (Jeremiah 17:7-8)

(Jesus spoke), "I am the true vine, and my Father is the gardener. [2] He cuts off every branch in me that bears no fruit, while every branch that does bear fruit, he prunes so that it will be even more fruitful. [3] You are already clean because of the word I have spoken to you. [4] Remain in me, as I also remain in you. No branch can bear fruit by itself; it must remain in the vine. Neither can you bear fruit unless you remain in me.
[5] "I am the vine; you are the branches. If you remain (or abide) in me and I in you, you will bear much fruit; apart from me you can do nothing. [6] If you do not remain in me, you are like a branch that is thrown away and withers; such branches are picked up, thrown into the fire and burned. [7] If you remain in me and my words remain in you, ask whatever you wish, and it

will be done for you. ⁸This is to my Father's glory, that you bear much fruit, showing yourselves to be my disciples.
⁹"As the Father has loved me, so have I loved you. Now remain in my love. ¹⁰If you keep my commands, you will remain in my love, just as I have kept my Father's commands and remain in his love. ¹¹I have told you this so that my joy may be in you and that your joy may be complete." (John 15:1-11)

Reflect on the way water is drawn from the roots, through the vine and into the branches. Why do you think Jesus refers to himself as the "true vine"?

How is bearing fruit the proof that the branch is connected to the vine? What does a branch do to bear fruit?

What does the Father do to the branch that bears no fruit? What does He do to the branch that does bear fruit?

What pruning has God done in your life, and what fruit have you seen as a result?

How many times is the word "remain" mentioned in the passage?

How does Jesus describe what remaining (or abiding) in him looks like and what are the results of abiding in him?

Chapter 7
The Potter and Clay

The potter/clay imagery is mentioned many times in the Bible to describe God's work of shaping and molding our character and lives. The Great Potter easily shapes and works with clay that is pliable and yielding, rather than clay that is tough and hardened. Our Creator, whose love is supreme, and whose plans are only good, intends to shape and mold us into the person of his design.

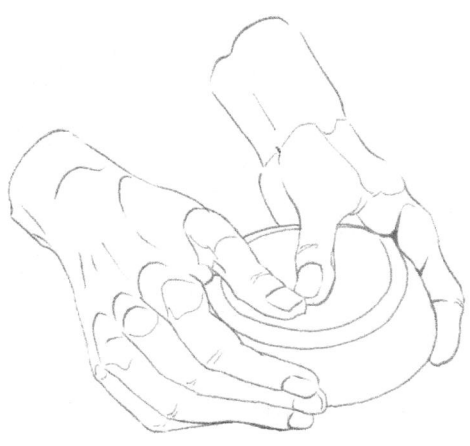

While living in Turkey years ago, I experienced the unique process of pottery-making up close upon visiting the quaint town of Avanos, one of the pottery centers of Anatolia. It sat on the Kizil Irmak (or Red River), the banks of which provided the rich red mud for the artisans to use on their potter's wheels.

I was mesmerized as I walked into several shops laden with red pots of all different shapes and sizes, as well as a variety of multicolored vases, plates, jugs, and bowls, painted with all kinds of geometrical designs. The sound of the artisans slapping the mud on their whirling wheels filled the air. I watched one skilled artisan add water and then press and knead the clay on his wheel while constantly turning the base with his feet.

He explained how he used his sensitive touch and slightly angled his finger or palm to shape the clay as it spun. He also explained how important it was to carefully shift the angle of both hands together to achieve a symmetrical and smooth shape to the final product. All this while spinning the base with his feet! True to his culture and hospitality, the friendly potter offered me his place at the wheel and insisted I try it out. He had made it look so easy; I assumed it couldn't be that difficult!

As I tried in vain to spin the base of the wheel with my feet while working on the clay with my hands, I realized the years of experience and mastery it took to achieve the level of skill this artisan had reached. Furthermore, my hands had simply not achieved the sensitivity or control needed to shape the clay. I stared at my asymmetrical and lumpy bowl, which was a pitiful sight on the wheel. I couldn't help but humbly ask the master potter to come back and rescue my mud blob to reshape it into something beautiful!

Surrender to the Master Potter

Humbly yielding to God and the asking him for courage to trust him as he shapes our hearts and character are an essential part of the transformation process. Yielding our will in submission to his can be painful because of the hopes and dreams we so tightly hold on to. Trusting God for our lives is not something that comes naturally to our human nature! However, he is the Master Potter and knows exactly what he's doing. The secrets and intents of our heart are deep, and he knows how to shape them and develop our soul and character in a way that will have lasting effect and eternal significance. Left to our own devices, we make a mess of things, just as I did with my clay blob. With a bit of work, kneading, water added, and more spinning, the Turkish potter had shaped up my clay into a beautiful vase in no time.

At key times in my life, I wrestled with God. I was hard clay, not yielding to his shaping and molding in my life. I found it difficult to trust him with my hopes and dreams for the future. During my twenties and thirties, as the years raced by as a single, I found it difficult to yield my hopes for marriage to him while living in countries where life as a single woman was challenging, and prospects for marriage were slim.

Years later, after God brought me a wonderful husband, I then found it difficult to yield to him my hopes for children. I faced years of infertility and grief and the very real possibility of never being able to have kids. I wrestled with God over both these dreams and gradually learned to trust him to do whatever he saw best, in his way and time. The trials were painful, yet shaped my character and made me learn to trust him more. My character and relationship with him developed in a way that couldn't have been achieved without the trials. Experiencing his faithfulness in my past trials helped me face the cancer journey with confidence and assurance of his sovereign love and work in my life.

~Reflect~

Yet, you, Lord, are our Father. We are the clay, you are the potter; we are all the work of your hand. (Isaiah 64:8)

Like clay in the hand of the Potter, so you are in My hand...but they reply, "It's no use. We will continue with our own plans; we will all follow the stubbornness of our evil hearts." (Jeremiah 18:6,12)

But we have this **treasure** in jars of clay to show that this all-surpassing power is from God and not from us. (2 Corinthians 4:7)

We are God's **masterpiece**. He has created us anew in Christ Jesus, so we can do the good things he planned for us long ago. (Ephesians 2:10)

You turn things upside down,
   as if the potter were thought to be like the clay!
Shall what is formed say to the one who formed it,
   "You did not make me"?
Can the pot say to the potter,
   "You know nothing"? (Isaiah 29:16)

What words are used in 2 Corinthians 4:7 and Ephesians 2:10, to describe us, the work of God's hands?

Imagine clay that hardens and is unyielding in the potter's hands. How do our attitudes and hearts become like unyielding clay in God's hands?

What does he want us to do when this happens?

Are you soft or hard clay in his hands? Why?

Write out a prayer asking God to make you soft clay in his hands and help you yield to his shaping in your life.

Chapter 8
The Good Shepherd and Sheep

"I am the good shepherd. The good shepherd lays down his life for the sheep."
-Jesus in John 10:11

As a good shepherd painstakingly cares for his sheep no matter the weather conditions or threat to his own life, so Jesus wants to be our shepherd and tend to our needs wholistically. God is depicted numerous times in the Old Testament as a shepherd caring for His people. This analogy is carried over into the New Testament by Jesus in John 10 when he declares he is the Shepherd: "I am the good shepherd; the good shepherd lays down his life for the sheep." That is exactly what he did. The Messiah God gave his life as a sacrifice in substitution for ours when he died in our place on a Roman cross.

The Dreaded News

The shepherd/sheep imagery was the first thing to come to mind after receiving the dreaded news. "It is cancer." The phone call came on a Friday afternoon in August, earlier than I expected. I had the biopsy just the day before and didn't anticipate the results until Monday, so my heart skipped a beat when I glanced at my buzzing phone and saw it was my doctor.

After dashing upstairs to take the call privately, I was already out of breath, so to hear "It is cancer" took what was left of my breath away! Suddenly, I felt like a truck had just hit me, and I was speechless. It took the rest of the afternoon to calm down and adjust to this devastating news. Just two weeks before, I had celebrated my fifty-fifth birthday. My family told me I was in "such good shape" and "looked a decade younger." Indeed, I did feel great and enjoyed walking, running, tennis, and many other activities. Being a registered dietitian, I had always valued nutrition and a healthy lifestyle. The cancer news certainly shattered whatever sense of invincibility I had, assuming these healthy habits could somehow guarantee that I'd be shielded from cancer!

John 10 filled my mind, allowing me to calm down and think again. Specifically, it was the verse, "The good shepherd lays down his life for the sheep... ." Jesus, my shepherd, already laid down his life for me. He's given me everything. I have nothing to fear, even death itself. The reality of his love, his plans, his promises, and past faithfulness in my life had built an unshakable foundation. Therefore, when this news came, a profound peace and sense of his presence and sovereignty enveloped me at the same moment. I was ready for whatever kind journey I was to embark upon. That's when I remembered "La Mano Del Arenal," the hand statue from Costa Rica. God had already been preparing me for this!

Psalm 23 is one of the most familiar and quoted passages of Scripture. Because of its familiarity, we overlook its many profound ideas and applications, which W. Phillip Keller's insightful book, *A Shepherd Looks at Psalm 23,* spells out.

The details of his job as a shepherd relate to each of the verses of the Psalm. In verse 1, "The Lord is my Shepherd, I shall not want," Keller, a real-life shepherd, contrasts his own well-provided for sheep with those of an irresponsible tenant shepherd, whose sheep are "thin, weak, and riddled with disease and parasites."[6] This is similar to the idea Jesus presents in John 10. There, Jesus describes the tenant shepherd, or "hired hand" as abandoning the sheep, and running away when he sees a wolf attack, "...he is a hired hand and runs away because he cares nothing for the sheep" (John 10:12, 13). The one whose shepherd is Christ finds a foundational security based on his promises to care for her soul and body. After processing the shock of my cancer diagnosis, God gave me inner strength and a renewed joy as I prayed though the verses of Psalm 23.

~Reflect~

Pray with me, or formulate your own prayer based on Psalm 23:

The Lord is my shepherd, I lack nothing.
>   He makes me lie down in green pastures,
> he leads me beside quiet waters...
>   he refreshes my soul.
> He guides me along the right paths
>   for his name's sake. (Psalm 23:1-3)

"Lord, you are my shepherd, and you perfectly take care of me. You knew about the cancer from the time it started, and you have a sovereign plan for good. You are my strength and all I need. My relationship with you is the solid rock of my life and I will not be shaken. Your love, power and authority in my life is greater than death or disease. You hold my cancer in your hands, and I trust you; I will not be in want. You have not withheld anything good from me.

I ask you to make me lie down in green pastures of hope and encouragement, feeding on your promises and enjoying your presence during this trial; that your word will be my bread each day and your truth my sustenance. I trust you to still my soul and deliver me from fretting and anxiety that threatens to overwhelm me.

Lead me beside quiet waters, refresh my soul and make me look only to you in dependence at this time. For your name's sake, be glorified and honored in this trial."

> Even though I walk
>   through the darkest valley,
> I will fear no evil,
>   for you are with me;
> your rod and your staff,
>   they comfort me. (Psalm 23:4)

"Lord, I have no idea how bad this cancer really is, how much it has spread, or if it's metastasizing through my body. You know it completely and are in control. I ask you to heal me, stop the growth, and eradicate it completely. I can trust you fully as I surrender this uncertainty to you, trusting you with all my life. Even if death is the outcome, I trust you with my family, my husband, and kids that you will provide their needs. As I walk through this dark valley, you are reigning over my life, and you will accomplish everything that concerns me and each of my family members. Make this cancer serve your greater purposes and higher plans. Deliver me from fear and anxiety."

You prepare a table before me
   in the presence of my enemies.
You anoint my head with oil;
   my cup overflows.
Surely your goodness and love will follow me
   all the days of my life,
and I will dwell in the house of the Lord
   forever. (Psalm 23:5-6)

"Lord, you will supply my physical, mental, emotional needs even as the enemy tries to accuse, blame, or cast doubt. You have won the victory over the evil one and all his attacks against me. You are for me, and your plans are good, you provide me a future and hope, all the days of my life, and I will always be with you now and for eternity. Your goodness and love will be with me. Thank you for your promise that I will always dwell with you."

For further reflection, look up John 10:1-21 in a bible or online and read about Jesus' teaching of himself as our shepherd. List your observations here.

Chapter 9
Trust and Surrender

The prayer based on Psalm 23, which I prayed that Friday afternoon, was one of surrender and trust. When we open our hearts and hands of prayer, we can imagine them labeled *trust* on one and *surrender* on the other. The two literally go hand in hand!

Over the weeks of waiting for appointments, scans, and test results, God built up my faith muscles of trust and surrender through daily practice. I often felt overwhelmed with anxiety and had to constantly return to the Shepherd in prayer, holding fast to his promises in his word. The act of trust and surrender is never a onetime practice but a daily habit and activity in which God trains us.

Elisabeth Elliot, one of my favorite authors and life examples, was a woman who knew well the path of suffering and loss and had a lot to say about surrender. She entered the Ecuadoran jungle with her young daughter to live with and translate the Scriptures for the Waodani people, an Amazonian tribe that had murdered her husband and four other missionaries. Her well-known story, *Through the Gates of Splendor*, tells of how she waited on God, surrendered, forgave, and courageously followed God's call. Years later, she remarried and lost her second husband to cancer. She refers to these and various other trials in her book, *A Path Through Suffering*, in which she describes this posture of surrender and openness to God:

> Open hands should characterize the soul's attitude toward God—open to receive what he wants to give, open to give back what he wants to take. Acceptance of the will of God means relinquishment of our own. If our hands are full of our own plans, there isn't room to receive his.
>
> The outer leaves of a flower make up what is called the calyx. Like tiny hands it clasps the bud, holding tightly to the furled petals, but as the flower develops the hold is

loosened, though still maintaining the power to contract. In maturity there is a complete release, a letting go, and the mini- hands are folded back, past all power of closing. [7]

God fills opens hands that are surrendered to him. Only those hands which are empty, holding nothing back, can receive what God intends to give. We may disagree with him about what is best, but this is where trust comes in: that we believe he is good. We willingly release our wishes while receiving his better plan for us, even though it may bring suffering.

Elisabeth Elliot also wrote, "One does not surrender a life in an instant. That which is lifelong can only be surrendered in a lifetime." [8] I had to give over my future and the anxiety of my cancer diagnosis daily, affirming through prayer my trust in him no matter what happened.

Elliot further wrote about surrender: "Leave it all in his hands that were wounded for you." [9] Who best to give over our concerns and future to but the one who loves us most, who died for us, and who is the God of the universe? Trust and surrender take a great deal of willpower—the directing of our will toward whatever God has for us rather than what we wish for ourselves. It involves sacrificing our will on the altar and agreeing with God that his sovereign plan for us is better—even if it's more difficult or painful. With the cancer diagnosis, the cross of Christ had indeed cut across my will to the point where I had to surrender my future, my family, and the uncertainty of my diagnosis to his sovereign will and love.

Through surrender we don't fight or argue with God or allow bitterness or self-pity any entrance into our hearts. During my cancer battle, many scripture passages at that time greatly helped me to maintain an open heart to trust God and receive from him. They reminded me that God has wonderful goals in mind for the trial I was going through. God wastes none of our tears or heartache but has a good plan for each. "You keep track of all my sorrows. You have collected all my tears in your bottle. You have recorded each one in your book" (Psalm 56:8, NLT).

~Reflect~

No discipline seems pleasant at the time but painful. Later, however, it produces a harvest of righteousness and peace for those who have been trained by it. (Hebrews 12:11)
Note: Discipline in this verse of Hebrews 12:11, is *paideia* in Greek, referring to all that's included in child-rearing, like training, education, instruction, chastisement, and correction. The idea of this verse is that God is training us, such as a good parent trains a child, or a coach trains an athlete. Through God's custom training program, He helps us toward reaching full development and maturity in Christ.

Consider it pure joy, my brothers and sisters, whenever you face trials of many kinds, because you know that the testing of your faith produces perseverance. Let perseverance finish its work so that you may be mature and complete, not lacking anything. (James 1:2)

For our light momentary troubles are achieving for us an eternal weight of glory that far outweighs them all. So we fix our eyes not on what is seen, but on what is unseen, since what is seen is temporary, but what is unseen is eternal. (2 Corinthians 4:17, 18)

Therefore, I urge you, brothers and sisters, by the mercies of God to present your bodies as a living and holy sacrifice, acceptable to God which is your spiritual service of worship. (Romans 12:1)

Cast your cares on the Lord, and he will sustain you, he will never allow the righteous to be shaken. (Psalm 55:22)

Cast your anxiety on him because he cares for you. (1 Peter 5:7)

Jesus says, "Come to me, all who are weary and heavy-laden, and I will give you rest." (Matthew 11:28)

You will keep in perfect peace those whose minds are steadfast,
because they trust in you. Trust in the Lord forever,
for the Lord, the Lord himself, is the Rock eternal. (Isaiah 26:3, 4)

May the God of hope fill you with all joy and peace as you trust in him, so that you may overflow with hope by the power of the Holy Spirit. (Romans 15:13)

Trust in the Lord with all your heart
    and lean not on your own understanding;
in all your ways submit to him,
    and he will make your paths straight. (Psalm 3:4-6)

Based on the previous Scriptures, what are some things God promises to do through your cancer trial?

What does he promise us as we trust him?

What does trusting God look like in your cancer trial? What are ways he is asking you to trust him?

In your cancer trial, how is God training you to grow in maturity as we see in Hebrews 12:11?

~Pray~

"Heavenly Father, I know you don't waste anything, and you have a purpose in my cancer diagnosis. As I go through this trial, help me trust you to make the "eternal weight of glory" (2 Corinthians 4:17) greater than the temporary suffering I experience. I present my body to You as a holy sacrifice. I give you my thoughts, attitudes, wishes, test results, and the concern of the cancer spread. I am weary of bearing the burden of these worries and cast these cares on you. Jesus, I receive your rest and the sustaining grace and joy of fellowship with you as I go through this. Thank you for your care and love for me which is perfect and greater than that of any human being. I can trust You fully, no matter what the future holds. Whether it's good or bad news, I praise you ahead of time and accept your sovereign decisions. Use my diagnosis for Your glory and purposes."

Chapter 10
Anxiety

"Be to me a rock of habitation to which I may continually come; You have given commandment to save me, for you are my rock and my fortress."
-Psalm 71:3

Taking my concerns to him in prayer daily was incredibly stress-releasing. He did indeed prove to be a Rock of habitation to which I could continually come each day. However, despite all this, a level of anxiety persisted that threatened to rise up like a wave and wash over me. After prayers of surrender and trust, I struggled with having to address it again and again.

Remember, the process of praying through our anxiety and trusting Christ is a daily posture and activity God is shaping in us. This continual reliance upon God creates an intimacy and fellowship with him that God has designed as we look to him in dependency. I was reminded of the simple prayer Jesus taught his disciples: "Give us this day our daily bread" (Matthew 6:11). This means *daily* coming to Christ for our needs. The "bread" mentioned here is God supplying our spiritual as well as our physical needs. Jesus refers to himself in John 6:35 as the bread of life. "Then Jesus declared, 'I am the bread of life. Whoever comes to me will never go hungry, and he who believes in me will never thirst.'"

God urges us in Psalm 68:19 to come to him daily for our needs and concerns: "Blessed be the Lord, who daily bears our burden, The God who is our salvation." God wants to deliver us from anxiety, which if not dealt with, drains our soul, sucking life out of us. "Anxiety weighs down the heart" (Proverbs 12:25). Don't be surprised that we need to go to Jesus many times throughout the day to receive his peace and find release from anxiety.

I never felt in my journey that I "conquered" anxiety completely or that it was a settled issue. But through the process of needing to continually return to him, I realized he had developed in me the behavioral and attitudinal reality of dependency on him. He calmed my heart, pouring out his peace each time I prayed and sought his presence. Spending time in the Psalms and other scripture and praying them back to God is an especially good way to receive from him and allow him to build a solid foundation of his peace and truth in our life.

Walking with Peace Through the Sea of Anxiety

God often has us walk this parallel path of both deep peace and nagging anxiety, just as the Israelites did when God led them to freedom through the Red Sea in the book of Exodus. The walls of water were held back at God's command, and the Israelites walked through on dry land. They were safe and secure, yet the walls of water surrounding them must have been terrifying as they journeyed through the night. Despite fear, they believed God's promise and proved their belief by walking through the sea. Yet, their precarious reality remained; they were completely vulnerable, surrounded by walls of water that would destroy them all if God did not protect them. For the long hours it took them to cross, their journey was indeed a parallel path of anxiety and peace. For them, the pillar of fire and smoke (Exodus 13:21), which was always present, reminded them that God was with them in the midst of their anxiety.

Likewise, though we don't see a pillar of smoke, we must remember that God is with us always when He has us walk our own parallel paths of peace and anxiety. The path of trusting God through cancer is a secure and solid path, even though we still struggle with our fears. Anxiety is not eliminated, but we are not controlled by it, since our anchoring is in Christ and his sovereignty and lovingkindness.

Keeping to the path of peace was a particular struggle for me. During the first six to eight weeks when the diagnosis and cancer spread was not completely certain, I spent a lot of time waiting to get in to see specialists, have MRI's, schedule surgery, and get back test results. I constantly had to go to the Lord to ask him for help and strength to walk in his peace and not become overwhelmed by anxiety. It all took time and lots of waiting, which I longed to hurry up and be done with. Yet, at this most anxious time, he caused me to experience his peace and filled me with joy, praise, and a renewed perspective on my life. It was evident to me during this time that he caused me to live on a plane of peace that was beyond my own capacity.

The Reality of Uncertainty and Being Out of Control

Living with the uncertainty of a health threat such as cancer is stressful, but the reality is, we don't know what tomorrow will bring whether we have cancer or not. God used my cancer diagnosis to make me understand I had already been living in uncertainty yet had not realized it. The veneer of being in control is deceptive. We live in a delusion that we are in a secure and certain world of our own making and ignore the fragility and uncertainty of where our life can take us at any moment.

As it says in the book of James, "Come now, you who say, 'Today or tomorrow we will go to such and such a city, spend a year there, buy and sell, and make a profit." Yet you do not know what your life will be like tomorrow. You are just a vapor that appears for a little while and then vanishes away" James 4:13,14 (NAS).

In view of the reality that we are utterly dependent upon God for every breath and each day we live, what else can we do but yield to his dealings with us in faith and dependency, resting in the palm of his loving and sovereign hand as he holds us securely in himself?

~Reflect~

I sought the Lord and he answered me and delivered me from all my fears. (Psalm 94:19)

For I am the LORD your God, who upholds your right hand,
Who says to you, 'Do not fear, I will help you.' (Isaiah 41:13)

So do not fear, for I am with you; do not be dismayed, for I am your God. I will strengthen you; I will uphold you with my righteous right hand. (Isaiah 41:10)

Cast your anxiety on him because he cares for you. (1 Peter 5:7)

Do not be anxious about anything, but in every situation, by prayer and petition, with thanksgiving, present your requests to God. And the peace of God, which transcends all understanding, will guard your hearts and minds in Christ Jesus. Finally, brothers and sisters, whatever is right, whatever is pure, whatever is lovely, whatever is admirable-if anything is excellent or praiseworthy-think about such things. (Philippians 4:6-8)

God has not given us a spirit of fear, but of power, love, and self-control. (2 Timothy 1:7)

For you have not received a spirit of fear leading to slavery again, but you have received a spirit of adoption as sons and daughters, by which we cry out Abba Father. (Romans 8:15)

From the prior verses, what are some of the reasons why God says we are not to fear or be anxious?

In Romans 8:15, what does a spirit of fear lead to, and what does God want to give us instead?

In 2 Timothy 1:7, what kind of spirit does God want to give us?

In Philippians 4:6-8, what does it look like to "present your requests to God"?

Looking at 1 Peter 5:7, how do you think the word *cast* helps us understand the idea of giving something over to God?

Looking at Philippians 4:6-8, what are God's instructions concerning our thought life? How do these new mental habits free us from anxiety?

~A Prayer Based on the Prior Scriptures ~

"Jesus, the wall of anxiety feels like it will crash over me. I need your peace and power to overcome my worries concerning the uncertainty and the unknown. Help me surrender the outcomes of my tests, results, and questions to you. Take my hopes and dreams. I lay them before you; take and receive them and let my hope be in your sovereign love and plans for my life, not my own hopes. Take my family members and give me assurance that you will take care of each one. I will not anxiously look about me, for you are my God. You will strengthen and uphold me with your righteous right hand. Fill me with thanksgiving and your peace that passes all understanding to guard my heart and mind. Let your consolations be my delight. Thank you that you are my Helper, I will not fear. I cast my cares on you because you care for me. Take my anxious thoughts and let your presence be my peace. Thank you that I am redeemed by Jesus' blood and sacrifice on the cross and have been adopted in your family. You are my Abba-Father. I reject fear and receive your power, love, and self-control. You have not given me a spirit of fear which results in slavery to anxiety, but you have given me your Holy Spirit, and as your daughter/son,

I trust in you to do what is best in my life as you determine it. Thank you that "He who did not spare his own Son but gave him up for us all-how will he not also, along with him, graciously give us all things" (Romans 8:32)."

Chapter 11
Disease or Dis-ease?

New Paradigms and Priorities

Have you ever had a radically different way of looking at things, which suddenly confronts your habitual way of thinking and doing? We may call this a paradigm shift. As I sat at the dinner table that Friday evening after learning of my diagnosis, I was still wrestling with anxiety and wondering when my husband and I should break this news to our kids. Yet, as I glanced at each of my family members, I felt an overwhelming sense of gratitude for each one and for that moment I had with them. The reality of the value of my relationships and the gift of the present time struck me in a new light.

In the weeks following, what birthed in me was a new view of the present time and an awareness of enjoying and living in the moment. Along with this was an urgency to make better use of my time for the eternally significant. Moments became gifts. Time and days revealed their inestimable value. Thanks to God's grace, I had undergone a very welcomed and beneficial paradigm shift.

It's interesting that the word *disease* was written as *dis-ease* prior to the 16th century and simply meant "lack of ease or comfort, rather than a medical illness." [10] God showed me that he was using this disease of cancer, creating a state of "dis-ease" in the old sense of the word, to move me out of my comfort zone of ease and into a new paradigm of fresh gratitude and purpose.

Evaluating Present Activities and Time Priorities

How is God using your cancer to help you move out of your comfort zone of "ease" and into new paradigms and priorities he's planned for you? Reflect on the well-known prayer of St. Augustine, "Our heart is restless, O Lord, until it finds its rest in you." Our cancer can be a tool in God's hands to help us reevaluate the eternal purposes of what we are living for and help us ache for the eternally significant. Are our present activities, pursuits, and ambitions leading us to build God's kingdom, rather than pursuing our own self-interests, and will they result in God's honor and glory that will last in eternity?

The Eternal and the Temporary

The reality of this very temporary time we call "life on earth" compared to eternity came crashing in on me after receiving the cancer diagnosis. Suddenly, the temporary yet urgent concerns and pressures of my schedule shrank to their true size. I became more keenly aware of the eternally significant actions and pursuits which God wanted me to focus on. With this renewed vision and God's guidance, I focused my attention upon practical ways to share his love and word with others around me. The value of time with others became more tangibly important and of transcendent meaning. In general, I noticed myself slowing down, letting go of the insignificant (yet seemingly urgent things), allowing balls to drop that really didn't matter anyway, and live life more simply and deliberately focusing on the eternally significant.

Is the disease of cancer moving you toward dis-ease in a life-giving, transformative way? Is it moving you into new patterns, priorities, and activities, some of which may be out of your comfort zone? Ongoing transformation as we follow Christ will start with the heart and work itself outward affecting our actions and behavior. Let your disease be the "dis-ease" that moves you into the healthy paradigm shifts and priorities He has designed for you.

~Reflect~

For I am about to do something new. See, I have already begun! Do you not see it? I will make a pathway through the wilderness. I will create rivers in the dry wasteland. (Isaiah 43:19, NLT)

Stand at the crossroads and look; and ask for the ancient paths, ask where the good way is, and walk in it; and you will find rest for your souls. But you said, 'We will not walk in it.' (Jeremiah 6:16)

But seek first his kingdom and his righteousness and all these things will be added to you. (Matthew 6:33)

Then you will know the truth, and the truth will set you free. (John 8:32)

... pursue righteousness, godliness, faith, love, perseverance, and gentleness. (1 Timothy 6:11)

Do not conform to the pattern of this world but be transformed by the renewing of your mind. Then you will be able to test and approve what God's will is-his good, pleasing, and perfect will. (Romans 12:2)

He has shown you, o man, what is good. And what does the Lord require of you? To act justly and to love mercy and to walk humbly with your God. (Micah 6:8)

Love the lord your God with all your heart and with all your soul and with all your mind and with all your strength ... and your neighbor as yourself. (Mark 12:30, 31)

Then Jesus came to them and said, "All authority in heaven and earth has been given to me. Therefore, go and make disciples of all nations, baptizing them in the name of the Father and of the Son, and of the Holy Spirit, and teaching them to obey everything I have commanded you. And surely, I am with you always, to the very end of the age." (Matthew 28:18-20)

According to the prior verses, what are the priorities God gives us to focus on?

Which of these had you never thought of before?

What are you hearing from God about what he wants you to do?

Write out a prayer based on the above verses and answers you've written.

Chapter 12
Distractions

Paradigm shifts, fresh vision, and new priorities don't last unless they are maintained as a lifestyle habit. It's easy to get caught up in the "tyranny of the urgent" and become like ants scurrying around, busy but not accomplishing the new priorities and mindset God wants us to focus on.

Coming Back to True North

Balancing the necessary things to do in life while maintaining this eternal perspective is difficult. With a cancer diagnosis thrown in, life and logistics become that much more complicated. My time with God has always been the daily habit that keeps my compass directed to True North. During this time with God, as we read his word and pray, our minds refocus on the eternal and are renewed by meditating on his promises. Self-destructive attitudes are corrected, and ideas for loving others are inspired. We hear from Jesus and experience the joy of fellowship with him.
This time with God may differ in form, place, and duration depending on the changing seasons of life. However, making time for him is important because it will serve as one of the habits by which we receive God's blessing, grace, and truth in our lives to help us follow him. In Luke 10:38-42, we see Jesus emphasizing this truth that being at his feet and listening to him is one of the most necessary activities in our lives. He commends Mary, who "chose what is better." That is, she chose to sit at Jesus' feet to listen and learn from him with a quiet heart rather than rushing around trying to meet the expectations of others or finishing tasks on her to-do list.

> [38] As Jesus and his disciples were on their way, he came to a village where a woman named Martha opened her home to him. [39] She had a sister called Mary, who sat at the Lord's feet listening to what he said. [40] But Martha was distracted by all the preparations that had to be made. She came to him and asked, "Lord, don't you care that my sister has left me to do the work by myself? Tell her to help me!"

[41] "Martha, Martha," the Lord answered, "you are worried and upset about many things, [42] but few things are needed— or indeed only one. Mary has chosen what is better, and it will not be taken away from her."

We have many tools to help us focus on Jesus during our time with him. One of the most helpful habits I have found is to simply keep a notebook and write short notes of the Scripture passages I read to track what God is saying to me through his word. At the same time, if distracting thoughts or unfinished tasks come to mind, I jot them down so I can get to them later, freeing me from distraction in order to listen to God.

In my notebook, I use a simple method of asking, "What does the passage say, what does it mean, and how can I apply it to my life?" After reflecting and writing these things, I pray over all I've written. Highlighting and underlining verses is a great way to assimilate, review, and remember them later.

Bringing the Lord into the daily activities of our work, daily tasks, and medical appointments is another great way to connect with God. When responsibilities don't demand our full attention, we can turn our thoughts back to praying and connecting with God, perhaps by listening to the Bible on audio, reading over our journal notes from our time with him, praying for those around us, or thanking and praising him. As Brother Lawrence, a monk from centuries ago, stated in his classic *The Practice of the Presence of God,* "My only prayer practice is…I carry on a habitual, silent, and secret conversation with God that fills me with overwhelming joy…in the noise and clatter of my kitchen, while several persons are at the same time calling for different things, I possess God in a great tranquility as if I were on my knees." [11]

Attending to our daily work and tasks naturally prevents us from focusing on the connection we have with God. However, by returning our minds to him during breaks, we can keep that channel open. Furthermore, we too can learn the "secret," as Brother Lawrence did, of maintaining peaceful fellowship with God amid the "noise and clatter" of our tasks and activities.

Distraction Pitfalls

For most of us, the time-consuming distractions of online news, social media, and a barrage of emails and texts pose one of the greatest threats to a heart at rest in God's promises. Setting boundaries like silencing our phone, turning it off in the evenings, or limiting social media, are all great ways to avoid digital distraction. Reading the Bible and life-giving books, pursuing hobbies, volunteering in our community, and connecting face to face with friends, rather than diving into the digital world, are key ways to connect with others and God.

As we go through our cancer journey, sharing what we are experiencing and learning with a friend is one of the most healing and refreshing things we can do. This strengthens our faith, builds up others, and gives us a connection of influence as we relationally share and receive. Depending on personality and how we are feeling physically during our cancer or treatments, this can be easier for some than for others.

Also, it's easy to distract ourselves searching online for support groups or spending lots of time researching the latest medical interventions. These things may seem to give a temporary peace but can never fill the gap in our hearts, which only the foundational and lasting peace of Christ can provide. We continually read in the New Testament of God's design for face-to-face relational encounters that provide real connections through which his love flows from one person to another in true fellowship. Consider the following scriptures:

Therefore encourage one another and build up one another, just as you also are doing. (1Thessalonians 5:11)

Therefore comfort one another with these words. (1 Thessalonians 4:18)

...that I may be encouraged together with you while among you, each of us by the other's faith, both yours and mine. (Romans 1:12)

But encourage one another day after day, as long as it is still called "today," so that none of you will be hardened by the deceitfulness of sin. (Hebrews 3:13)

In his book *12 Ways Your Phone is Changing You*, Tony Reinke makes the point that "Digital distractions keep thoughts of eternity away.... We find it easy to fall into the trap of digital distractions, because in the most alluring new apps, we find a welcome escape from our truest, rawest, and most honest self-perceptions. Distractions give us easy escape from the silence and solitude whereby we become acquainted with our finitude, our inescapable mortality..." [12]

Our "finitude" and "inescapable mortality" are the places where God wants to meet us. If we let them, digital distractions rob us of the joy of connecting with God and others at these moments. Rather than turning our minds and hearts to him, through connecting with him in his word and in prayer, we can easily fill them with the candy of internet fodder or digital entertainment. Tragically, these can keep us from the rich and life-giving relationships with God and others that he's provided to satisfy our souls. In addition, some content and images we take into our minds from certain movies, books, and other media can impede our moving forward towards Christlikeness and the abundant life.

~Reflect~

Do not be deceived, God is not mocked; for whatever a man sows, this he will also reap. (Galatians 6:7)

Finally..., whatever is true, whatever is honorable, whatever is right, whatever is pure, whatever is lovely, whatever is of good repute, if there is any excellence and if anything worthy of praise, let your mind dwell on these things. (Philippians 4:8)

We are destroying speculations and every lofty thing raised up against the knowledge of God, and we are taking every thought captive to the obedience of Christ. (2 Corinthians 10:5)

And do not be conformed to this world, but be transformed by the renewing of your mind, so that you may prove what the will of God is, that which is good and acceptable and perfect. (Romans 12:2)

And this I pray, that your love may overflow still more and more in real knowledge and all discernment, so that you may approve the things that are excellent, in order to be sincere and blameless until the day of Christ. (Philippians 1:9,10)

Make a list of actions God wants you to take according to the previous Scriptures.

What does he want us to set our minds upon?

Why are thoughts, thinking patterns, and habits so important for transformation?

Write out a prayer based on the previous verses and answers you've written.

Chapter 13
Soul Healing Under the Great Surgeon's Knife

Days stretched into weeks of waiting. After the first shocking news of hearing the word "cancer," it took time to schedule and complete all the necessary appointments and tests to finally have the surgery. These included trips to the oncologist, the cancer surgeon, the plastic surgeon, pre-op appointments, an MRI, more blood tests, and an EKG. Eight weeks passed from the time I got the shocking news of the cancer to when it was finally removed through a left mastectomy. Those were a very long eight weeks. At times, I felt distressed, realizing the cancer was alive and well, growing, and possibly spreading throughout my whole body! As I anticipated the arrival date of the surgery, I prayed often, asking God to prevent the spread of the cancer during the waiting period.

The Malignancy of Sin

Now, the idea of someone wanting to hurry up and have a mastectomy is absurd except in the context of cancer. The knowledge of a growing, life-threatening, aggressive tumor makes all the difference in one's attitude to undergo such a surgery. It makes us eager and willing to yield to the surgeon's knife to accomplish ultimate healing. In this context, we clearly see the deadliness of our disease and the need to have a clean break and freedom from the malignancy.

Weeks before the surgery, I was yearning to have it out as quickly as possible. I hated having to wait, wondering if it was growing and spreading. During that time, I compared my anticipation to have the surgery to what our attitude about the cancer of sin should be when we finally realize its malignancy and destructiveness to our soul and life. It made me reflect on how Jesus cut off and forgave my sin years ago when He came into my life and how thankful I was that He dealt with this Cancer of Soul, the epidemic of all mankind.

Facing Sin

In our human nature, sin is something we often want to excuse, ignore, or rationalize. Even the word *sin* seems archaic to modern ears, but it simply refers to doing what God desires us not to do and not doing what He wants us to do. It is also the self-seeking mindset of directing and living our lives without God. Romans 3:23 says, "All have sinned and fallen short of the glory of God."

Not one of us can meet the perfect standard of righteousness needed to have peace with God in a righteous relationship with him. It says in Isaiah 59:2, "Your iniquities have separated you from your God; your sins have hidden his face from you, so that he will not hear." The Greek word for sin is *hamartia*, which literally means *missing the mark*, as an arrow misses its center mark on a target.

If we knew how malignant and metastatic sin is to our soul, emotions, and life, we would eagerly want to go under the Great Surgeon's knife to have it removed. Sin blinds and deceives. It causes a callousness of heart that shuts out God's light and the work of his Spirit to point it out and deliver us from it. Like a malignant tumor, our sin is a relentlessly growing force of destruction. I often recalled this illustration of the "tumor of sin" as I was waiting to have the surgery.

Whose Standard?

We all have our own standard of righteousness or morality, or how we define right and wrong. We form our understanding of what sin and righteousness are from our family of origin, our culture, experiences, and beliefs. Our conscience is vital in our personal assessment of right and wrong and developing our moral law. C.S. Lewis points out that our conscience and observance of a natural law is one of the pieces of evidence of God's existence and one way God communicates with us. Our conscience helps us know when we have transgressed our moral law. In fact, our conscience and personal set of standards point to the existence of an ultimate Law Giver.[13]

We all have a sense of a moral law, which is influenced by our presuppositions. As Francis A. Schaeffer observed, "Most people catch their presuppositions from their family and surrounding society, the way that a child catches the measles. But the people with understanding realize that their presuppositions should be chosen after a careful consideration of which worldview is true." [14] Many of us simply absorb a worldview, rather than carefully choosing it. It's like asking a fish to describe what it's like to be wet!

Only as we come to understand God's moral law can we see the errors of our own presuppositions and worldview.

God's Perfect Standard: Jesus and His Teaching

The ultimate revelation of God's perfect standard is Jesus himself, the incarnation of God in human flesh Who dwelt among us. He lived and walked perfectly in obedience, righteousness, and love upon this earth. John 1:1 and 14 describe this: "In the beginning was the Word, and the Word was with God, and the Word was God… And the Word became flesh and made his dwelling among us. We have seen his glory, the glory of the one and only Son, who came from the Father, full of grace and truth."

Furthermore, in Jesus' teaching, particularly the Sermon on the Mount in Matthew chapters 5-7, He explains God's perfect standard of morality by covering many topics common in life including: Interpersonal relationships, facing conflict, honesty, hypocrisy, handling anger and reconciliation, receiving and giving forgiveness, sexual purity, loving others, prayer, fasting, finances, dealing with anxiety, authentic faith, and purpose in life. Look up Matthew chapters 5, 6, and 7 in a Bible or on the internet. As you read, use a pen and paper to write a list of man's ideas of righteousness in one column and a list of God's standards of righteousness in another. This makes for a good study to clearly see the difference between our idea and God's idea of "good."

We can easily overlook how God views these different areas of life which we experience daily. The Sermon on the Mount is one of the most life-giving teachings of Scripture because in it we find ourselves caught with his flashlight on the hidden places of our heart. If we are honest, we have to agree with God about the discoveries of prejudice, judgment, pride, self-will, lust, greed, and the chasm between our concept of righteousness and his. Like a cancer diagnosis, the truth, which was previously hidden, is revealed. The bad news must be revelatory before we can find healing. We have no place to go but to the Great Physician and under the Surgeon's knife for the healing of our soul.

God Looks on the Heart

From the Sermon on the Mount and many other passages in Scripture, we understand that Jesus focuses on the heart. It all begins with the heart, the seat of the mind, will, desires, and ambitions. This is the part that God seeks to change and transform. Jesus' sacrifice and payment for our sin satisfies God's righteous requirement of a death payment. "The wages of sin is death but the gift of God is eternal life in Christ Jesus our Lord" (Romans 6:23).

"Death" in this verse refers to death physically, spiritually, and relationally as sin causes us to be separated from God. Jesus' death on the cross and his resurrection from the dead save us from the destructiveness of our sin and our own self-seeking way. This redemptive work of Christ brings us into a right relationship with God. He sends his spirit into our hearts and minds to make us one with him so that he can begin transforming us into the image of his Son, if we ask him. Following Jesus is impossible without the work of Christ in our hearts to cause rebirth and provide ongoing grace and power from his Holy Spirit that dwells in us after we believe. This is why the Bible says, "All have sinned and fall short of the glory (or perfect standard) of God" (Romans 3:23), and "Unless you are born again, you cannot see the Kingdom of God" (John 3:3).

A Deeper Look at the Broken Image

In our human tendency, it's natural to believe we are basically "good enough" to achieve a right standing before God. Many religions have the idea of a scale, where the good and bad deeds are weighed, and if your good deeds outweigh your bad, you're in! However, God's standard, not ours, is what matters. He uses his standard of righteousness when the final day of accountability comes.

The Bible teaches we are made in God's image, but this image has been broken. Like a mirror, once able to reflect beautifully the face looking into it, our soul is marred by cracks and lines due to its brokenness. Deep down, we all know we are made for Something, Someone, and Somewhere better, but sin in our hearts makes each of us pursue our own way of fulfillment. As a result, we all seek independence from God in our unredeemed state. The mirror, our soul made in God's image, remains cracked. Although we see glimpses of the beauty of God in our lives, it's unrecognizable compared to the clarity and definiteness of its original state.

This happened in the fall of man in the garden in Genesis 3 with ongoing effects through the generations, resulting in the broken image of every individual. However, God's love and compassion for us did not let him leave us in our broken states. His solution for our soul healing and restoration is in his Son, sent to us in human flesh, who paid a debt he didn't owe for sinners who couldn't pay.

When we believe in him and receive his solution for our sin problem, we become one with Christ. In this oneness with Christ, God sees his righteousness in us and our sin on him. This mystery of new birth is explained in the verses: "God made him who knew no sin to be sin for us, so that in him we might become the righteousness of God in him" (2 Corinthians 5:21), and "We all like sheep have gone astray, each of us has turned to his own way; and the Lord has laid on him (Jesus) the iniquity of us all" (Isaiah 53:6).

~Reflect~

All have sinned and fall short of the glory of God. (Romans 3:23)

We all like sheep have gone astray, each of us has turned to his own way; and the Lord has laid on him (Jesus) the iniquity of us all. (Isaiah 53:6)

If we say we have no sin, we deceive ourselves and the truth is not in us. (1 John 1:8)

The heart is deceitful above all things and beyond cure. Who can understand it? (Jeremiah 17:9)

You know that he appeared in order to take away sins; and in Him there is no sin. (1 John 3:5)

God made Him who knew no sin to be sin for us, so that in Him we might become the righteousness of God. (2 Corinthians 5:21)

Do not let sin reign in your mortal body so that you obey its lusts. (Romans 6:12)

But your iniquities have separated you from your God; your sins have hidden his face from you, so that he will not hear. (Isaiah 59:2)

If your right eye causes you to stumble, gouge it out and throw it away. It is better for you to lose one part of your body than for your whole body to be thrown into hell. And if your right hand causes you to stumble, cut it off and throw it away. It is better for you to lose one part of your body than for your whole body to be thrown into hell. (Matthew 5:29, 30)

Put on the Lord Jesus Christ and make no provision for the flesh in regard to its lusts" (Romans 13:14).

Whoever is in Christ is a new creation, the old has passed away, the new has come. (2 Corinthians 5:17)

Therefore, as you have received Christ Jesus the Lord, so walk in Him, rooted and built up in Him and established in the faith, as you have been taught, abounding in it with thanksgiving. (Colossians 2:6, 7)

Believe in the Lord Jesus and you will be saved. (Acts 16:31)

Yet to all who did receive him, to those who believed in his name, he gave the right to become the children of God. (John 1:12)

He saved us, not because of righteous things we had done, but because of his mercy. He saved us through the washing of rebirth and renewal by the Holy Spirit. (Titus 3:5)

What are some of the destructive consequences of sin?

Based on the previous verses, write a definition of sin.

What is God's remedy for our sin?

How are faith and repentance (turning from sin to God) related?

The First Step in Following Jesus

A drowning person has no hope of life unless someone intervenes and reaches down to deliver him from sinking to his watery death. In the same way, if you have never experienced God reaching down to save you from drowning in your sea of sin and self, I encourage you to seek him and ask him to do this work in your life. Praying a certain prayer itself is not what brings us forgiveness, rather it is turning to Christ, in simple faith, believing in him for salvation and forgiveness of sins as you trust him to transform you through his Spirit.

~Pray~

"Dear God, thank you that you died for me, and Jesus' sacrifice is the perfect and sufficient payment for my sin, which I could never begin to pay for. Without your sacrifice, your sinless life given for me, the sinner, I would truly drown in my sins without any hope of eternal life with you. Jesus, thank you that by your resurrection you have conquered my sin and death and offer me life in yourself. Please reach down and rescue me from my sin and self to follow you. Give me the gift of your Holy Spirit to help me walk with you each day."

Chapter 14
Turkish Carpets, Canvases, and Suffering

While living in Turkey, I bought a Turkish carpet that sits in my house today and is full of memories from the time I lived there, including the experience of buying it! I can still picture the colorful shop packed with hundreds of carpets hanging, folded, and stacked on every shelf and in every corner. Immediately upon my entering, the shopkeeper asked countless questions to determine my style and colors of interest. With one motion of his hand, his two helpers instantly sprang up from their stools and hurriedly rushed to retrieve carpets of various sizes and patterns. Turkish tea was quickly ordered, a chair pulled out, and I was asked to sit down, get comfortable, and watch the "show."

I stared with delight as each flick of their wrists caused the carpets to quickly unroll in ripples of waves, revealing seas of design and color. The shopkeeper talked nonstop, giving detailed explanations for the symbols and patterns of each unique design. After about half an hour of this flurry of unfurling and persuasion, I finally reached a decision. My carpet bore the classical Ottoman design in the middle with threads of blue, white, grey, black, and red woven in intricate patterns to create a beautiful geometric and floral design around the sides. These were machine-made carpets, and like their handmade counterparts, were uniquely designed beforehand with the finished product in mind.

Custom Made by a Master Designer

Our Master Designer also knows ahead of time what he is weaving in our lives. He knows the patterns, unique experiences, and trials, that have shaped our personality, character, and ways of relating to him and others. These are unique and special to us as our fingerprints. Several times in Turkey, I was able to watch the fascinating process of handmade carpets being woven on large upright wooden looms, where the back as well as the front can be clearly observed.

The back of the carpets resembled a chaotic jumble of threads with no organization and provided no clear way to guess what the front pattern would look like. Oftentimes our own lives can seem as disharmonious as the backs of carpet. This is often true when we look at it from the side of our human perspective. However, God sees the true perspective from his side. We can trust him even when he allows the darker threads of suffering and pain to be woven in. The darker threads are often the ones needed to emphasize and set apart a pattern or differentiate a unique shape, giving the carpet its crowning touch. When I struggled through the shock of my cancer diagnosis, this carpet illustration came to me in a fresh new way and reminded me of the purposefulness of suffering in God's economy.

The Designer is working hard to blend and put together the unique shapes, patterns, and colors which He's planned. Each thread matters to him. In the dark thread of suffering, we can rest assured and even rejoice that God is working hard to create a masterpiece. C.S. Lewis emphasized the purposefulness of pain in his work *The Problem of Pain*, in which he compares God to a master artist at work on a canvas:

> We are, not metaphorically but in very truth, a Divine work of art, something that God is making, and therefore something with which He will not be satisfied until it has a certain character. Here again we come up against what I have called the "intolerable compliment." Over a sketch made idly to amuse a child, an artist may not take much trouble: he may be content to let it go even though it is not exactly as he meant it to be. But over the great picture of his life—the work which he loves, though in a different fashion, as intensely as a man loves a woman or a mother a child—he will take endless trouble—and would doubtless, thereby give endless trouble to the picture if it were sentient. One can imagine a sentient picture, after being rubbed and scraped and re-commenced for the tenth time, wishing that it were only a thumbnail sketch whose making was over in a minute. In the same way, it is natural for us to wish that God had designed for us a less glorious and less arduous

destiny; but then we are wishing not for more love but for less. [15]

God takes "endless trouble" to arduously work on the canvases of our lives. Let us yield to his work and wish for more, not less of his "glorious destiny" and design for us.

My perspective on suffering has also been helped by reading several of Joni Eareckson Tada's books over the decades. Having had a diving accident at the age of seventeen, not only has she spent most of her life with quadriplegia, but she has endured her own cancer journey and has much to say about suffering. However, she has not let suffering stop her from living a full life. The author of over forty books, Tada also creates beautiful artwork with her mouth, recorded several musical albums, advocates for people with disabilities, and is the founder and leader of the ministry *Joni and Friends*. In an interview, she commented, "I'd rather be in this wheelchair knowing God than on my feet without him." She reflects in her writing, "My weakness, that is my quadriplegia, is my greatest asset because it forces me into the arms of Christ every single morning." And "... here I sit ... glad that I have not been healed on the outside, but glad that I have been healed on the inside. Healed from my own self-centered wants and wishes." [16]

~Reflect~

For this momentary light affliction is preparing for us an eternal weight of glory, beyond all comparison, as we look not to the things that are seen, but to the things that are unseen. For the things that are seen are transient, but the things that are unseen are eternal. (2 Corinthians 4:17-18.)

For I consider the sufferings of this present time are not worthy to be compared with the glory that is to be revealed to us. (Romans 8:18)

Therefore, since we have been justified by faith, we have peace with God through our Lord Jesus Christ. Through Him we have obtained access by faith into this grace in which we stand, and we rejoice in the hope of the glory of God. Not only that, but we rejoice in our sufferings, knowing that suffering produces endurance and endurance produces character, and character produces hope, and hope does not put us to shame because God's love has been poured out into our hearts though the Holy Spirit who has been given to us. (Romans 5:1-5 ESV)

All discipline for the moment seems not to be joyful, but sorrowful; yet to those who have been trained by it, afterwards it yields the peaceful fruit of righteousness. (Hebrews 12:11, NAS)

According to the prior verses, how does God want to use the suffering and affliction we go through?

Suffering can make us bitter or better. How do we react in a way so God will use it to make us better?

Write a prayer based on the above verses and answers you've written.

Chapter 15
The Powerful Effect of Thanksgiving

The first few weeks felt like a bombardment of bad and shocking news:

"Suspicious calcifications," read the mammogram report.

"Invasive carcinoma," read the biopsy report.

"Mastectomy," said the cancer surgeon.

"Chemo is a likely treatment followed by radiation," said the oncologist.

The looming decision as to which route to take with my breast reconstruction added to my stress. Certain options would have to be implemented in my upcoming mastectomy surgery, with completion in subsequent surgeries. I had very little time to learn all I needed to know to make this complicated decision.

The Attitude of Gratitude

Over those first few months, I felt weighed down with the thought of surgeries, chemo, and radiation, but the biggest concern was the cancer itself. Was it spreading? My husband and I waited eagerly to hear about the initial MRI results. Finally, I got the anticipated call from my cancer surgeon that according to the MRI, it appeared no cells had spread to the surrounding lymph nodes. That would be confirmed later with a pathology report after surgery.

The good news brought us relief and opened my eyes to God's provision and mercy not to allow the cancer to spread despite the size of the tumor and who knows how long it had been there! This brought me into a perspective of thanksgiving that transferred to many other areas of life and helped set the pace for gratitude during my whole cancer journey. God was teaching me to be grateful for every piece of good news, every blessing, and every provision of his in their various forms.

Offer Thanksgiving and Praise to God

God also used this perspective of gratitude to help me express thanksgiving and praise to him for all things, good or bad. The days afterward were filled with both positive and negative reports, including the reality that I would indeed have to go through chemo. Through it all, I felt God had picked me up and put me into a new dimension of thankfulness and joy that were beyond circumstance. He caused me to see every blessing as a true gift of his, whether it was my family, friendships, good health, or the peace of resting in his care. Likewise, I was learning to give thanks for his future provision of grace and strength in facing chemo, radiation, and surgeries down the road. As I grew in living with the perspective of thanksgiving, even the tough decisions surrounding the reconstruction seemed less weighty.

The Right Perspective Enhances Thanksgiving

About the same time, I had a couple of God-ordained conversations with various individuals, which God used to help me with this perspective of thanksgiving. At a rehab center where I worked as a registered dietitian, I met a patient who had just gone through a leg amputation. He had an amazing attitude despite the challenges he was going through. God brought to my attention that I have two healthy legs, and losing a breast will not hinder me from mountain hikes, biking expeditions, tennis matches, or other things I enjoy!

With this perspective, I took time to experience gratitude and give thanks for my health overall and the ability to stay active. By reflecting on what I did have and giving thanks for what I had previously taken for granted, God taught me to walk in a lifestyle of thanksgiving and joy.

My greater awareness of God's gifts grew into a path of joy and wonder. These gifts included not only good medical care but relationships, provisions for basic needs, and the great outdoors. Even some tasks I considered quite mundane became sources of thankfulness!

> He brought me up out of the pit of destruction, out of the miry clay; And he set my feet upon a rock, making my footsteps firm. He put a new song in my mouth, a song of praise to our God; Many will see and fear and will trust in the Lord. (Psalm 40:2,3)

Walking in Thankfulness

As the journey grew into weeks and months, challenges came with surgery, chemo, and radiation, which threatened to thwart the "attitude of gratitude" that had powerfully set me on a course of joy. However, God showed me along the way that the very things I wanted to complain about were loving provisions from him. One of these was the tissue expander, placed during my mastectomy surgery to stretch the skin and make room for the reconstruction at a later surgery. Another was my chemo port, placed several weeks later to receive chemo infusions at a faster rate than a normal IV. Both were uncomfortable and intrusive and took time to get used to. Before surgery, a friend who'd experienced the tissue expander advised me not to focus on it being there.

With some time for healing and keeping my thoughts away from the tissue expander and the port, I came to a place of contentment with these two devices. Since my reconstruction surgery was delayed due to chemo and radiation, I ended up having the tissue expander fourteen months longer than I expected. Making "gratitude lists" and praying through them in praise to God were great ways to solidify the attitude of gratefulness as a reality in my mindset. After the first several weeks of recovery, I hardly thought of the tissue expander, and unbeknownst to me, it turned out to be the best preparation for my unexpected implant surgery later.

Thankfulness Despite Interrupted Plans

From the beginning, I had planned for a DIEP (or deep inferior epigastric perforator artery) flap reconstruction. In this type of autologous reconstruction, one's own tummy fat tissue is used in a transplant surgery wherein the patient is both the donor and recipient. Unfortunately, my ten-hour DIEP flap surgery failed, and I had to settle for plan B, an artificial implant.

After wrestling with insurance for months over the coverage for the DIEP flap and having high hopes that it would work and restore me to my most natural pre-mastectomy state as possible, I was incredibly grieved that it failed. Plan B, having an implant, was certainly not something I was looking forward to! Furthermore, I had read about cases of Breast Implant Illness (BII), where the body reacts to the implant and causes harmful side effects. I had talked personally with someone who experienced this, and it was a genuine concern. Nevertheless, throughout the fourteen-month period with the tissue expander, which includes an implant, I had none of the symptoms; therefore, I knew this would not be a concern for me. God used my experience with the tissue expander to put my mind at ease and make the mental adjustment to an implant much easier than it would have been otherwise.

After finishing chemo and radiation, I continued Herceptin infusions (a targeted immunotherapy treatment) for a year. I needed my port for these infusions, just as I did for chemo, so I ended up having the port for about a year longer than I had hoped! At times, when I tired of having the port, I was reminded of a family friend who went through chemo in Sarajevo, Bosnia, where he was not able to get a port put in for his infusions. Not only did the infusions last longer than mine, without the port to speed up the rate of infusion, but each time he went in, it became increasingly harder to find a vein. He'd been poked so many times that his veins became overused.

Suddenly I could not help but feel genuine gratitude for my port and the good health care I'd received. Around this time, I also watched a video series on the historical figure John Adams and saw the brutal portrayal of Adams' grown daughter undergoing a mastectomy-without modern anesthesia of course.

God used several similar situations to help me see his mercy toward me and to make me realize I had an immeasurable amount to be grateful for. Though we often take them for granted, modern technology, good health care, anesthesia, and effective treatments are God's merciful provisions many of us in advanced countries are incredibly fortunate to have today.

As G.K. Chesterton amusingly points out regarding the gratitude we easily overlook, "When we were children, we were grateful to those who filled our stockings at Christmas time. Why are we not grateful to God for filling our stockings with legs?" and in observing the effect that gratitude brings, "I would maintain that thanks are the highest form of thought, and that gratitude is happiness doubled by wonder." [17]

~Reflect~

I will give thanks to You, LORD, with all my heart; I will tell of all your wonderful deeds. I will be glad and rejoice in you; I will sing the praises of your name, O Most High. (Psalm 9:1)

Give thanks to the LORD, for he is good; his love endures forever. (Psalm 107:1)

He opens His hand, and he satisfies the desire of every living thing. The LORD is righteous in all his ways and merciful toward all that he has made. (Psalm 145:15-17)

Devote yourselves to prayer, keeping alert in it with an attitude of thanksgiving. (Colossians 4:2)

Through Him then, let us continually offer up a sacrifice of praise to God, that is, the fruit of lips that give thanks to His name. (Hebrews 13:15)

Let the peace of God rule in your hearts, to which you were called in one body; and be thankful. (Colossians 3:15)

...always giving thanks to God the Father for everything, in the name of our Lord Jesus Christ. (Ephesians 5:20)

...give thanks in all circumstances; for this is God's will for you in Christ Jesus. (1 Thessalonians 5:18)

Every good and perfect gift is from above, coming down from the Father of heavenly lights, who does not change like shifting shadows. (James 1:17)

According to the previous Scriptures, when do we give thanks to God? And what do we give thanks for?

Why does God tell us so often in Scripture to give thanks to him?

Why is God the focus of our thanksgiving?

List as many things as you can think of that you are grateful for, both tangible and intangible.

What things do you wish you were more grateful for?

Write down the things that are difficult to thank God for, especially what you want to complain about. Ask God to help you give thanks for these things and begin now to thank God for them. Continue this pattern when you face these challenges.

Chapter 16
Contentment

"The heart of man is restless till it finds its rest in Thee."
-St. Augustine

God continued teaching me surrender, trust, and thankfulness throughout my cancer journey. The fruit that sprang forth next in the progression was contentment. In the first months after receiving my diagnosis, I kept thinking that I wanted to "be done" with surgery and treatment as soon as possible and get "back to normal." I felt that to reach a place of contentment, I would have to get all this behind me and return to my normal state. The wonderful thing about God is that he doesn't let us stay in our "normal state!" He is always working on us and in us, as Philippians 2:13 states, "… for it is God who works in you to will and to act in order to fulfill his good purpose."

I saw God use the long process of the cancer journey to graciously work contentment and other Christ-like qualities in my life. At times I wanted to quit, fed up with ongoing treatments and tired of discomfort. However, God showed me he could use my weakness as a springboard for his strength and endurance. God helped me release these ongoing trials to him and be glad that he would provide the endurance and contentment I needed—not only to survive the long journey but to thrive in the quality of abundant life he intended.

Humility was a constant theme that kept coming up for me as I wrestled with discontentment and a complaining attitude. I knew I needed humility to receive the trial, be patient through it, and submit to him the timeframe and physical constraints brought on by cancer. Though this was often difficult, he kept pointing me to prayer to ask and receive from him the grace and endurance I needed. It was most often through reading the scriptures that he gave me the words and truth I needed to press on.

James 1:21 says, "…in humility receive the word implanted." A humble and meek posture toward God establishes the condition for his word to take root in our hearts and cause transformation and fruit, especially in the midst of a trial. The Greek word for humility in James 1:21 is *prauteti* from the root *praus* that means power under control, or a reserved strength. It carries with it the idea of a wild horse that has been tamed and finally becomes rideable. Prauteti is repeated numerous times in the Bible, where it is translated as patience, meekness, and gentleness.[18] So rather than wriggling out from under God's hand and short-circuiting the merciful work he wants to accomplish in our character, he helps us submit to what he wants to do in his timeframe, not ours. With the perspective of gratitude and the surrender of my timeframe for the journey, he worked contentment in me.

~Reflect~

I have learned to be content whatever the circumstances. I know what it is to be in need, and I know what it is to have plenty. I have learned the secret of being content in any and every situation, whether well fed or hungry, whether living in plenty or in want. I can do all this through him who gives me strength. (Philippians 4:11-13)

Humble yourselves, therefore, under God's mighty hand, that he may lift you up in due time. (1 Peter 5:6)

Pride ends in humiliation, while humility brings honor. (Proverbs 29:23 NLT)

Based on the above Scripture, write out a prayer asking God to help you humbly receive the timeframe for your cancer journey and treatments. Ask him to give you contentment and joy in the journey.

Chapter 17
Teatime with God

Spending time with God and receiving from him are crucial for growing in Christ during our cancer journey. Being in his presence while listening to him helps us focus our hearts and minds on his truth. During this time, as we open our hearts to God and sit in his presence, he communes with us. We allow him to search our hearts as we read his word and pray. Praise, confession, thanksgiving, and supplication (making requests) are all a part of this time.

As way of illustration, I am reminded of a colorful scene from years ago when I worked in Uzbekistan. I lived with an Uzbek family the first several months in the country, and the hospitable mother of the family was eager to explain the traditional tea ritual to me the first morning I was with them. The early morning sun streamed in through the window on the round loaves of bread, cream, yogurt, cheese, and fruit spread out on the breakfast table. Gesturing to a nearby cushion, she urged me, "Kelib O'tiring," or "Come and sit down."

After donning her brightly colored robe and head scarf, she carefully placed a beautiful, deep-blue ceramic tea pot on the low-lying table, next to where I sat on velvety cushions on the floor with the other family members. She tipped the teapot, pouring the steaming contents into one of the small cups.

With a beautiful wide grin, she declared in Uzbek this first cup of light green tea as "loy" or "mud." Lifting the lid, she poured the contents of the cup back into the pot. After a few more minutes of steeping and lots of chit chat in Uzbek, she repeated the same actions, declaring the second slightly darker cup as "moy" or "oil." After several more minutes and lots more stories and conversation, she poured a third darker cup, declaring it, "choy" or "tea." Just when I thought that concluded it, she repeated it a fourth time, for good measure, guaranteeing the tea was indeed worthy to be served and consumed!

Coming Back to Jesus

I saw the tea tradition repeated on many occasions while living in Uzbekistan and reflected that spending time with God in his word each day is a bit like the tea steeping in the teapot. Through engagement with God's

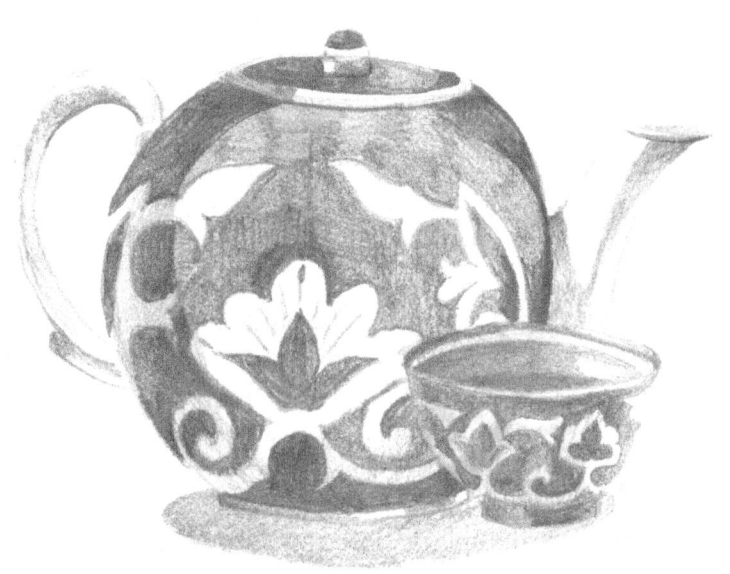

word and being immersed in it like the tea leaves in hot water, we are able to spend time in his presence and experience his life through us. Asking questions as we read, praying the Scripture in conversation with God, and hearing from him are all ways that help us engage with him in his word.

We often need to return to him for this "teatime." Just as the cups of tea were poured back into the teapot, we need to return to him and spend time in his word and enjoy his presence. By doing this, we are prepared to be used by him, to share his life through us, and to be poured out in service to others with the same life-giving presence we experience in him.

~Reflect~

Your word is a lamp unto my feet and a light unto my path. (Psalm 119:105)

O how I love your law! I meditate on it all day long. (Psalm 119:97)

I have hidden your word in my heart that I might not sin against you. (Psalm 119:11)

Do not conform to the pattern of this world but be transformed by the renewing of your mind. Then you will be able to test and approve what God's will is-his good, pleasing, and perfect will. (Romans 12:2)

But the Advocate, the Holy Spirit, whom the Father will send in my name, will teach you all things and will remind you of everything I have said to you. (John 14:26)

Finally, brothers and sisters, whatever is true, whatever is noble, whatever is right, whatever is pure, whatever is lovely, whatever is admirable-if anything is excellent or praiseworthy-think about such things. (Philippians 4:8)

Sanctify them by the truth; your word is truth. (John 17:17)

Jesus answered, "I am the way, the truth, and the life. No one comes to the Father except through me." (John 14:6)

Listen to my instruction and be wise; do not disregard it. Blessed are those who listen to me, watching daily at my doors, waiting at my doorway. For those who find me find life and receive favor from the Lord. (Proverbs 8:33-35)

Therefore, get rid of all moral filth and the evil that is so prevalent and humbly accept the word planted in you, which can save you. (James 1:21)

Let the word of Christ richly dwell within you, with all wisdom teaching and admonishing one another.... . (Colossians 3:16)

The Lord is near to all who call on him, to all who call on him in truth. (Psalm 145:18)

Do not be anxious about anything, but in every situation, by prayer and petition, with thanksgiving, present your requests to God. And the peace of God, which transcends all understanding, will guard your hearts and your minds in Christ Jesus. (Philippians 4:6)

Rejoice always, pray without ceasing, give thanks in all circumstances, for this is the will of God in Christ Jesus for you. (I Thessalonians 5:17, ESV)

This is the confidence we have in approaching God; that if we ask anything according to his will, he hears us. (1 John 5:14)

According to the previous scriptures, what are some of the ways God's word becomes a part of us?

According the previous scripture, explain the value of immersing oneself in God's word.

What instruction and promises does God give us about prayer?

Chapter 18
Joy in the Midst of Weakness

Anyone going through cancer can attest to the fact that weakness is an ongoing and constant part of the journey. Weakness takes different forms, whether it's physical, emotional, or mental. I keenly felt the weakness of bad chemo days, unexpected waves of lightheadedness, insomnia, dizziness, and headaches. I remember well the shock and anxiety of the diagnosis causing mental and emotional exhaustion. Then came the recovery from surgeries, utter dependency on others, changes in routine and activities, and a general reduced capacity, depending on the diagnosis and treatment regime. Physical changes like hair loss, weight loss or weight gain, and some lasting effects like lymphedema, neuropathy, and lingering pain. For some, there are treatments and effects that will last the rest of life. All of these challenges take their toll on our happiness, mood, and emotions.

The Bible is full of references about weakness and filled with examples of those who walked through it. God's word holds nothing back. It is filled with honesty about the doubts, emotions, failures, and weaknesses of every major figure mentioned in Scripture. One example is David, who was on the run from his enemies and almost killed multiple times. He experienced abandonment, humiliation, moral failure, and the tragic consequences of his sin. The Psalms are filled with his writings which are full of honesty, doubt, questions, as well as praise. He seeks God earnestly and asks him many hard questions as he struggles with him over many things. God calls him, a "man after his own heart" (1 Samuel 13:14).

David authored a large portion of the Psalms, a prayer and praise book for the Hebrew people as well as the church throughout history. The Psalms are full of expressions of praise alongside desperate and honest prayers springing up from human emotions and weaknesses David and others experienced. In Psalm 13:1-2, he feels forgotten and hidden from God: "How long will you forget me, Lord? Forever? How long will you hide from me? How long must I worry and feel sad in my heart all day? How long will my enemy win over me?"

Despite his frustration, David proclaims his faith in God in verses 5 and 6: "I trust in your love. My heart rejoices because you saved me, I sing to the Lord, because he has taken care of me." David has joy amid great unhappiness and weakness! Joy, the unshakeable and certain rock in a believer's life, is not crushed by external forces but is based on our relationship with God in Christ. Circumstantial happiness, in contrast, floats on a sea of chance and emotion, with seemingly no higher purpose to the suffering.

We also see the example of Paul, who constantly suffered for the gospel and yet had joy in the backdrop of weakness. In sharing the gospel, he encountered "beatings, imprisonments and riots... sleepless nights and hunger ..." and was made "sorrowful, yet always rejoicing; poor, yet making many rich; having nothing, and yet possessing everything" (2 Corinthians 6:3-10). Again, Paul states, "... He (Jesus) said to me, 'My grace is sufficient for you, for my power is made perfect in weakness.' Therefore (says Paul), I will boast all the more gladly about my weaknesses, so that Christ's power may rest on me. That is why, for Christ's sake, I delight in weaknesses, in insults, in hardships, in persecution, in difficulties. For when I am weak, then I am strong" (Corinthians 12:9-10).

True Joy

Joy and happiness are two different things. Joy, which is found in the abundant life Jesus calls us to, has no substitutes. Yet, we often ignore the joy that God wants to give and settle instead for the happiness that his gifts of health, travel, career, success, family, and other earthly pleasures temporarily provide. C.S. Lewis beautifully describes this greater joy that can be ours in Christ:

> Our Lord finds our desires not too strong, but too weak. We
> are half-hearted creatures, fooling about with drink and sex

and ambition when infinite joy is offered us, like an ignorant child who wants to go on making mud pies in a slum because he cannot imagine what is meant by the offer of a holiday at the sea. We are far too easily pleased. [19]

The joy of being in Christ and experiencing his abundant life is far greater than these temporary gifts, which are just shadows of the real joy of being in fellowship with him and of the eternal life yet to come.

~Reflect~

Consider it pure joy, my brothers and sisters, whenever you face trials of many kinds, because you know the testing of your faith produces perseverance. Let perseverance finish its work so that you may be mature and complete, not lacking in anything. (James 1:2-4)

In the same way, the Spirit helps us in our weakness. We do not know what we ought to pray for, but the Spirit himself intercedes for us through wordless groans. (Romans 8:26)

For we do not have a high priest who is unable to empathize with our weaknesses, but we have one who has been tempted in every way, just as we are—yet he did not sin. (Hebrews 4:15)

[7] But we have this treasure in jars of clay to show that this all-surpassing power is from God and not from us. [8] We are hard pressed on every side, but not crushed; perplexed, but not in despair; [9] persecuted, but not abandoned; struck down, but not destroyed. [10] We always carry around in our body the death of Jesus, so that the life of Jesus may also be revealed in our body. (2 Corinthians 4:7-10)

As the Father has loved me, so have I loved you. Now remain in my love. If you keep my commands, you will remain in my love, just as I have kept my father's commands and remain in His love. I have told you this so that my joy may be in you and that your joy will be complete. (John 15:9-12)

Jesus praying to the Father, "I am coming to you now, but I say these things while I am still in the world, so that they may have the full measure of my joy within them." (John 17:13)

Jesus instructed his disciples, "Until now you have asked for nothing in my name. Ask and you will receive, and your joy will be complete." (John 16:24)

Though you have not seen him, you love him; and even though you don't see him now, you believe in him and are filled with inexpressible and glorious joy. (1 Peter 1:8)

Though the fig tree does not bud and there are no grapes on the vines, through the olive crop fails and the fields produce no food, though there are no sheep in the pen and no cattle in the stalls, yet I will rejoice in the Lord, I will be glad in God my Savior. (Habakkuk 3:17,18)

But He said to me, "My grace is sufficient for you, for my power is made prefect in weakness." Therefore, I will boast all the more gladly about my weakness, so that Christ's power may rest on me. That is why, for Christ's sake, I delight in weakness, in insults, in hardships, in persecutions, in difficulties. For when I am weak, then I am strong. (2 Corinthians 12:9,10)

My flesh and my heart may fail, but God is the strength of my heart and my portion forever. (Psalm 73:26)

What are some of the weaknesses mentioned in the Scriptures above?

What truths do the Scriptures point to which are factual and don't change with circumstances?

How does this affect the attitude and hope of those who put their hope in the certainty of these truths?

What weaknesses are you facing in your cancer journey?

What truths in these scriptures can you hold on to that are sure and certain, not changing with circumstances?

Write out a prayer of thanks to God for the hope and strength he gives you because of these truths.

Chapter 19
Cancer ... a Platform to Help Others

From the beginning of the cancer journey, I knew God was opening a door and preparing me to share his love and his salvation with others. I began meeting many others who were going through chemo or radiation at the same time as me. And I had friends going through other types of crises that I could relate to better because of the trial and suffering I was experiencing. It's only when someone endures a similar path of suffering can that person honestly say, "I understand." One purpose of God in our suffering is to understand and impart his comfort to others.

The One Who Understands Us Perfectly

Ultimately, it is Jesus who understands us best. When we reflect on his death on a Roman cross, one of history's most brutal forms of torture and suffering, we know he did this for us. Jesus, the Son of God, God incarnate in the flesh, allowed himself to suffer explicitly for our sakes. He did this not only as the payment for our sin, but to understand our weakness and sufferings, and as God incarnate, truly call us his brothers and sisters. Jesus was "despised and rejected by mankind, a man of suffering and familiar with pain" (Isaiah 53:3). We see in the following verses that he fully understands us in our pain, weakness, rejection, and other forms of suffering we experience.

...because he suffered death, so that by the grace of God he might taste death for everyone. In bringing many sons and daughters to glory, it was fitting that God, for whom and through whom everything exists, should make the pioneer of their salvation perfect through what he suffered. Both the one who makes people holy and those who are made holy are of the same family. So Jesus is not ashamed to call them brothers and sisters. (Hebrews 2:9-11)

For this reason, he had to be made like them, fully human in every way, in order that he might become a merciful and faithful high priest in service to God, and that he might make atonement for the sins of the people. Because he himself suffered when he was tempted, he is able to help those who are being tempted. (Hebrews 2:17,18)

For we do not have a high priest who is unable to empathize with our weaknesses, but we have one who has been tempted in every way, just as we are—yet he did not sin. (Hebrews 4:15)

Son, though he was, he learned obedience from what he suffered. (Hebrews 5:8)

We see from these Scriptures that Jesus, taking on human form and dying on the cross after experiencing various other forms of suffering while living on the earth, understands us perfectly. He is the perfect example of suffering: trusting and obeying God through it, without sin, and being the only one who could take that rightful place on the cross as our sacrifice and then resurrect from the dead. Jesus truly understands suffering and can come to the aid of those going through it. Furthermore, Christ is affected by the pain and suffering the members of his body go through.

Tim Keller explains this idea that when Jesus, after ascending to heaven, appeared to Saul (or Paul as he would be known) in a vision, in Acts 9:4. Saul was the main instigator of persecution against Christians very early in the book of Acts. Jesus, in the vision asked Saul, "Saul, Saul, why do you persecute **me**?" Keller makes the point, "Here we see that Jesus so identifies with His people that He shares in their suffering. When they are hurt or in grief, so is He." [20]

~Reflect~

(Christ Jesus) Who, being in very nature God,
    did not consider equality with God something to be used to his own advantage;
rather, he made himself nothing
    by taking the very nature of a servant,

being made in human likeness.
And being found in appearance as a man,
   he humbled himself
   by becoming obedient to death—
      even death on a cross!

Therefore, God exalted him to the highest place
   and gave him the name that is above every name,
that at the name of Jesus every knee should bow,
   in heaven and on earth and under the earth,
and every tongue acknowledge that Jesus Christ is Lord,
   to the glory of God the Father. (Philippians 2:6-11)

(v.3) Praise be to the God and Father of our Lord Jesus Christ, the Father of compassion and the God of all comfort, (v.4) who comforts us in all our troubles, so that we can comfort those in any trouble with the comfort we ourselves receive from God. (v.5) For just as we share abundantly in the sufferings of Christ, so also our comfort abounds through Christ. (v.6) If we are distressed, it is for your comfort and salvation; if we are comforted, it is for your comfort, which produces in you patient endurance of the same sufferings we suffer. (v.7) And our hope for you is firm, because we know that just as you share in our sufferings, so also you share in our comfort. (2 Corinthians 1:3-7)

How is God described in 2 Corinthians 1:3?

What does he do for us as we go through suffering?

What does the passage tell us about our purpose in suffering?

What are his promises as we share in the sufferings of Christ in verse 5?

What gifts does God impart to us through our suffering that we can pass on to others?

What good things has he given you so far through your cancer trial that you can pass on to others?

It is amazing to think that we can also pass on to others the same hope, promises, and words of comfort that Jesus gives us as we go through suffering. Having cancer provides a unique opportunity to share Jesus' love and salvation with those who may not have experienced him yet. I can think back to multiple social occasions where people asked how my cancer journey was going. God used these opportunities to share the good ways he had met me with his grace and love in the midst of the trials. Only in eternity will we fully understand our effect on others as a result of our obedience to Christ and our words when we righty attribute the credit and glory to Him.

Always be prepared to give an answer to everyone who asks you to
give the reason for the hope that you have.
But do this with gentleness and respect. (1 Peter 3:15)

Because we loved you so much, we were delighted to share with you
not only the gospel of God but our lives as well. (1 Thessalonians 2:8)

Chapter 20
Others' Stories

This chapter contains a compilation of the cancer stories of some of my dear friends. Most went through their cancer journeys years before I had mine. Their transparency inspired my faith and courage even before starting my own journey. I am sure their stories will do the same for you.

Heather's Story
Finding Emotions to be a Window to a Deeper Walk with God

I was diagnosed with Anaplastic Large T-Cell Non-Hodgkin's Lymphoma cancer. It was an aggressive form, but I had an ALK-positive marker that made it receptive to chemotherapy. My lymph nodes were swollen below the diaphragm, which was also a positive sign for treatment.

The struggles I felt over the course of my cancer journey ranged from sadness to fear to anger to helplessness. The sadness was associated with putting my family through the anxiety of whether I would survive. I really struggled to tell my sons the full story of what was going on. They were fourteen and thirteen at the time I was diagnosed. I didn't want to cause fear or anxiety in them. But my husband reminded me that this was a faith journey for all of us. We had to let them lean on their own faith as much as we had to lean on God for our own.

Fear rose up at points both during and in the years after treatment that the cancer wasn't going away or was returning. Having always thought of myself as a logical person, I had to come to terms with the fact that my mind could play tricks on me. I could talk myself into feeling similar pains or symptoms to those I had felt leading up to my diagnosis. Anger popped up at points when something didn't go as planned. My port wouldn't work the way it was supposed to and often slowed down my treatment. My biopsy site wouldn't heal because of the chemo and at one point burst open with an infection. I was so angry that it was another thing I had to fight.

Probably one of the strongest struggles was helplessness. I am a doer by nature, and as time went on, I grew weaker with each round of chemo. I also had to isolate one week out of every three in a chemo round. I couldn't take care of things around the house like I typically did. I couldn't work at my job at the pace I wanted. Some days, all I felt like doing was lying in bed or sitting in a chair. I felt terrible that everyone around me had to pick up what I could not do.

God met me in all of this. More than any other time in my life, I began to embrace my emotions and see them as an indicator of what was really going on inside of me. A lot of my Christian experience often made emotions out as bad, that we can't trust them. But I found that if I didn't try to push them away, and simply leaned into them, then God and I could have an honest conversation about what I was wrestling with in my heart and mind. I stopped being afraid of feelings, instead seeing them as a window to a deeper walk with him.

One of my most treasured but hard experiences had to do with fear rising up. I began to embrace the words of Psalm 91, to find refuge under the wings of the Almighty. This idea that I could take refuge in him from the raging unknowns became a source of great peace. In my helplessness, I saw how much he loved me, not because of what I could do, but because I was his child that he loved and created. His love was not contingent on me getting my to-do list done; neither was the love of other people. I embraced the idea that they could love me even if I couldn't do anything for them.

During this time, I would sometimes burst out crying when someone told me they were praying for me. Never had I felt the depth of need for prayer like I did during that time. I was touched deeply that others were taking my needs to the God the Father on my behalf.

Another lasting gift from my cancer journey is an appreciation for silence and solitude. I remember the first time I had to go for a PET scan, and they told me I would need to sit in a dark room by myself for an hour without anything to do while the radioactive dye kicked in followed by another thirty-plus minutes of lying still in the PET scan machine. I remember thinking, "Wow, am I going to be okay with just me and my thoughts during that time if I don't take a nap?" But God began to show me that it was a wonderful opportunity to be with him and to pray for others. In the past, my mind wanted to jump all around, but he taught me how to be okay (not perfect!) with that silence and solitude that let me just be with him.

Jeremy's Story
Three God Moments and Questions

I was forty-four years old when I was diagnosed with Chronic Lymphatic Leukemia, and my kids were ten, eight, and six at the time. I was serving as a fulltime Christian worker in the mission field of Central Asia, leading several teams from the capital city. I had to return with my family to South Africa for treatment.

The doctor decided to put me on the highest level of chemotherapy and said it was fifty-fifty as to whether it would work. It was eight treatments, in a three-week cycle, with three bone marrow tests—at the start, at the fourth treatment, and at the end.

The chemo treatment would give me such nausea and sickness that for a week, I would just survive, then, by the second week, all my white blood cells had died, and I had no energy to do anything. By the third week, I felt like a human again and then started the process all over. I was really only living one week in every three.

Even more difficult than the physical challenge was the feeling of having no future. I could not think of the future or anything lying ahead, and that took all the life out of me. No more dreams, no more plans, nothing to look forward to in this life. Also, well meaning "faith healing" friends were on me about doing chemo and not having enough faith in God for healing. Many friends avoided coming to see me because they didn't know what to say to a young man with cancer.

During this painful time, there were three large "God moments" where he spoke into my situation. He used these truths powerfully in my life and perspective.

The first happened one morning as I lay vomiting, feeling the chemo in my veins and tingling in my feet and fingers from the effects. My body was drained, and I was in physical agony. I went to Jesus in prayer, asking Him, "Can you understand how I feel?" Previously, I'd wondered why it wasn't enough that Jesus was crucified-why He also endured being whipped with many lashes beforehand. The crucifixion alone achieved the atonement, yes. But the severe physical pain-at the highest level and for a sustained period, did have a purpose. He DOES KNOW our pain I realized, every pain, and he can empathize. This became an incredible truth for me.

My second God moment came another morning as I lay exhausted, unable to get up, with my body's immunity at its lowest. I asked God, why, at forty-four years old, was I in this terrible situation? He answered me that morning with a question: "How does this thing end? What are the possible outcomes? One, you die and come to be with ME forever, or two, you live and continue to serve ME and love those around you. Which of those outcomes are bad?"

I had to agree with God that, indeed, there is no bad ending in his kingdom, and either ending was a good one. From that moment I had peace and never questioned God again about the illness or worried about the outcome.

My third God moment happened a week after God revealed the "no bad ending" truth. I suddenly realized that my wife and kids were not in that equation. My wife, being a strong believer, would be okay, but what about my kids who so dearly needed a father?

"What about them?" I asked God. "What happens to them if I die?"

"Who is their father?" HE asked me.

"OK, I get it." I admitted to God.

He, indeed, is even more their father than I am, and he assured me that he would fully care for them. It was a deep moment of hearing him, trusting him, and knowing his hand was over my life and my family.

I am now twelve years in remission at age fifty-eight, giving praise to God and thankful for every day that I have to be a light for him here on earth.

Slavko's Story
Just Five More Years…

At the beginning of 2008, I was diagnosed with testicular cancer. I was not quite thirty-nine years old. I was a church pastor in Sarajevo, the capital of Bosnia and Herzegovina, and had many plans and obligations. My calendar was full of things that needed to be done immediately. After visiting the doctor and receiving the diagnosis, I realized that my priorities were wrong. I started thinking about the brevity and transience of life and realized that some things that seemed urgent to me were not important at all from the perspective of eternity. Likewise, some other priorities that I thought there would be time for, since life seems so long, were actually more urgent. That was the first lesson I learned from that difficult initial experience with cancer, which two years later had forgotten.

Although the diagnosis was shocking, I took it quite well because the prognosis was good. The cancer was detected on time, it was on the border between the first and second stage, and the doctor explained to me that after surgery and medical treatments the possibility of survival was quite high. The fact that my father and grandfather died of cancer in their late thirties was not encouraging, but since they were not believers; they didn't have the advantage of the prayers of fellow Christian. In addition to advanced medicine, I had God on my side. I asked our church, and all the Christians I knew to pray for me. Knowing that God was in control brought peace and comfort.

The operation went without complications, and afterwards the doctor prescribed a series of radiation. The first follow-up examinations were encouraging: the tumor markers returned to normal. The oncologist informed me that for the first three years after surgery and therapy, I should have checkups every three months, and for the subsequent two years every six months, after which time I would be declared cancer free. I regularly went for checkups and was grateful to God that he seemed to be changing that pattern that had been running through my family for generations.

As time went on, I didn't like the checkups and doctor's visits and couldn't wait for three years to pass! Just as these years were coming to an end, I had sudden pain and was misdiagnosed with a kidney stone. I lost three months treating a nonexistent stone while a tumor on a lymph node in my abdominal cavity grew until it reached the size of a fist, completely blocking my ureter. This time, the diagnosis was not timely; the tumor surrounded the vena cava and surgery was not possible. The prognosis was not good due to the impossibility of surgical removal of the tumor. The only option was to try chemotherapy, but the doctors were not too optimistic.

The chemotherapy treatments were difficult and exhausting for my body, and this time I was unwell not only physically but spiritually. I thought that God had forgotten me and that the end of this life was near. I did not worry so much about myself because I believe and follow Jesus, and I know that at the end of this earthly life I will go to eternity with God. However, I was responsible for the care of my wife and children. Our daughter and son were young (fifteen and eleven), and my wife was not employed. We had just started paying off a house loan, and I was afraid that they would be left without a roof over their heads. I gave up praying for myself and just prayed for them. I was very restless until God spoke to me in prayer. I didn't get an answer to my questions, but I felt that God was asking me something. "Slavko, do you really think that you love them more than I do?" After this the anxiety was gone, and I knew that no matter what happened to me, they were safe in God's hands.

Although the prayers of believers and messages of encouragement were helpful, I did not feel spiritually well. I read in the Bible, in Proverbs 24:10: "If you faint in the day of adversity, your strength is small." I realized that although I was a pastor who preached regularly on Sundays and led Bible studies and prayer meetings, deep down in my heart I was not in a good place. My faith needed to be reset. The first step towards spiritual recovery is to realize and admit to yourself that you are not in a good place. After that, things spiritually took a turn for the better.

After the first cycle of chemotherapy, a control MRI was performed. The doctors were surprised because the tumor had completely disappeared, and there was no trace of it. They didn't expect that, and neither did I. My family history said that men die in their late thirties, but God had a different plan for me. On the doctor's advice, I underwent all four cycles of chemotherapy, which I endured physically well, while also remaining spiritually well.

As I write this in 2024, sixteen years have passed since the first diagnosis and fourteen since the second. I have been cancer free for a long time and I no longer go for checkups.

I am grateful to God for changing the fate of my family and extending the days of my life. Nevertheless, I am now aware of the transience and brevity of life, and how important it is that we live the days that God has determined for us to live on this earth with quality and for his glory. A sign in my home, which I got from a friend who is a cancer survivor, says, "Do not count days, make days count." These words remind me of this truth as I often remember how fourteen years ago, I prayed to God to give me *just five more years* of life to pay off a house loan so that my family would not be without a roof over their heads. I am grateful to him not only for the five years, but many more on top of that.

Angela's Story
My True Source …

I stood frozen in my kitchen as I held the phone to my ear. I was listening to the flat voice of the emotionally detached doctor on the other line saying, "You have invasive breast cancer. We don't know the extent of it yet. You need to come into the office to discuss this further." Reeling, I tried to process the words that hung in the air.

The phone call ended, and I dropped to my knees. Memories of my husband dying of cancer years before washed over me. I had held him as he took his last breath ... releasing him that final time back to Jesus. I couldn't do this. I couldn't face this. Fear gripped my heart as tears streamed down my face, and I looked towards Heaven, searching out the One who knew all things.

Within moments, I heard his calm, gentle voice: "This will not end like your husband's story." I waited in the stillness and tried to grab hold of the lifeline he had just thrown me as I struggled to keep my head above water. But...what would the report be from the doctors? How bad was the cancer? Regardless, my soul was stayed on his words: "In his hand is the life of every creature and the breath of all mankind" (Job 12:10). He brought an anchor as well in Psalm 139:16: "All the days ordained for me were written in your book before one of them came to be." He was the One clearly in control of this story, and he would be my keeper, no matter what happened.

I was a widow in my early forties, living alone, working full time as my only income. I had high hopes of still being remarried and having children one day soon. Dreams seemed to shatter on every front. Uncertainty was all around. They wanted to begin chemo immediately. They wanted to take both breasts after months of chemo. Only in that breast surgery, they told me, would they finally be able to stage the cancer and see its extent. Radiation would possibly follow. I would lose my hair by day twenty-one after starting chemo. My body would be forced into menopause and likely never come out of it to bear children.

I looked in the mirror at myself and touched my long, chestnut-brown hair that would soon be gone. My body would never look the same, and I grieved the loss of what I couldn't give my next husband. I wouldn't even be able to walk back up the three flights of stairs to my apartment after my surgery without help. The world spun around me as I clung desperately to Jesus.

The doctors said I should be grateful for my life: triple positive breast cancer ten years prior was terminal. They had no treatment then. So, I was given "life" somehow through the brutal drugs that seeped into my veins for eight hours every three weeks. My body revolted in every possible way until I begged the doctor, "No more! Please, not another round!"

It had been a long five months. My bald head was covered with a wig. Neuropathy had set into my feet, which were numb, and they weren't sure it would reverse. The high levels of prednisone I needed to endure the terrible side effects of chemo made me ravenous. I could not fit into the clothes that I reached for as I got dressed for work—on the days I could even go to work.

The time for the dreaded double mastectomy had come. Before I was wheeled away for surgery that morning, my closest friends gathered around my bed and offered up earnest prayers for my healing. The surgeon had slipped in while they were praying and quietly listened in the corner with prayers being said over him as well. I remember waking up in the hospital bed after surgery and searching the eyes of those who were beside me. Was it in the lymph nodes? Had the cancer spread? Comforting words met me: No lymph nodes. No spreading. They were able to get the cancer removed. And my prognosis was very good. I sank back in the bed with waves of gratefulness and worship. Yes, my body was altered, but my life had been spared.

Herceptin would continue for a year through the port they had built in my chest, but I tolerated it well. Reconstruction surgery was planned and would yield incredible results. Radiation was ruled out since the lymph nodes weren't involved. The extra weight quickly dropped off. I came out of menopause so rapidly, it shocked the medical staff. Coworkers donated their vacation time to cover all the days of work I had to be out. My wigs so closely matched my natural hair that most hadn't even realized I had lost my hair. Friends brought meals and gift cards. Bills were miraculously covered. My seventy-year-old parents came faithfully every three weeks to walk me up those flights of stairs and take care of me for days after each round of chemo. He *had* provided. He *was* providing. He *would* always provide.

Though we may sing sweetly on a Sunday morning about Jesus being our all and all, the rubber hits the road once "everything" is ripped away. I quickly realized through this deep valley that we can only surrender to the level we have been tried and tested. And I was at a whole new level. I simply could not know how much of my identity or confidence were in certain things or people or hopes for the future ... until I lost them.

WHERE was my source? WHO would be my true source? The Lord began to whisper to me and teach me. John 15 came alive to a level I never knew: "I am the Vine: you are the branches. If you remain in me and I in you, you will bear much fruit: apart from me you can do nothing." When you have nothing left, you quickly realize how many "things" have filled that gap that he alone should have filled.

He reminded me clearly as I looked down at my body, and out at my life and future, that HE was my Source. He began to walk me through what it looked like—and felt like—to be sourced in anything other than him. Yes, he gives good gifts for us to enjoy on this earth. Yet, if we go beyond the boundaries of what he has fashioned them for, THAT was "sourcing" ourselves in something else besides him.

Today, most people would never guess the journey I went through almost ten years ago. Yet, I bear the marks. Marks in the physical, but greater marks in the spiritual, of learning to source myself fully in him. Life on this earth with or without cancer is heartbreaking and full of pain. How good it is when we trod a well-worn path to the True Source where we can find relief! Grace. Peace. Joy. Strength. For ourselves and to share with others.

That is my prayer for you, dear reader, that through whatever you are facing today, you will know him as your True Source for all things: your greatest love, your healer, your provision, your hope. He will not waste a bit of your journey. Let him fill you to overflowing like only he can do. He has purpose in your story ... every chapter. Let the Author of Life write on your pages today the story of his glory shining through your situation!

Suzette's Story
I Would Not Trade the Trial

One summer evening in 2015, while cooking dinner for my husband and three young children, I prayed a very short prayer confessing that I needed to pray more faithfully for my children. My next prayer came about an hour later after I was greeted by an emergency medical technician in the ambulance on the way to my local hospital. The EMT explained with such kindness and care that I had had a grand mal seizure in my kitchen and that I would soon have tests done in the hospital to try to determine its cause. As I stared at the back door of the ambulance, Psalm 139: 11-12 came to my mind: "If I say, 'Surely the darkness shall cover me, and the light about me be night,' even the darkness is not dark to you: the night is bright as the day, for darkness is as light with you." I felt his peace and knew I was not alone. If he wasn't afraid, I didn't need to be fearful either.

Within a couple of days, an MRI and biopsy revealed I had an incurable, malignant brain tumor, and according to the doctor who diagnosed me, it was inoperable. Thankfully, my very resourceful husband sent my MRI scans to a few other reputable cancer treatment facilities for a second opinion. Each doctor confidently reported that a majority of the tumor could be surgically removed. We scheduled surgery right away with my new doctor whose role as a surgeon was to perform the surgery, but it was God who did the real work.

As soon as my mom saw the doctor after the surgery, she asked if he had been able to get the ninety-five percent of the tumor out that he said he thought he could remove. He said with a smile, "Let's just see what the radiologist report shows." That report revealed that all the tumor had been removed. We went from a doctor saying zero percent could be removed to another doctor getting 100% of it out!

After I recovered from the surgery, I started daily radiation treatments that lasted for a month. During my radiation appointments, I memorized and then meditated on Isaiah 41:10: "Fear not, for I am with you; be not dismayed, for I am your God; I will strengthen you, I will help you, I will uphold you with my righteous right hand." Believing his promise never to leave nor forsake me kept me full of peace.

Over the course of the year, I was going for regular MRIs every three months and each scan was showing that there was no new cancer and that my brain was healing nicely from the surgery. My oncologist was so encouraging and thorough. The doctors were hopeful that a successful surgery coupled with radiation treatment and one year of chemotherapy would lead to a better prognosis.

During this time of treatment, my family, friends, and various acquaintances, even strangers were providing meals, car rides, and help with various household tasks. My mom was an especially close and wonderful support. I was strengthened and encouraged by the spiritual and emotional support she gave daily.

I battled throughout each day to trust God with my life. We did not know if the treatments would kill the microscopic cancer cells. Would I live one year, three, five? No one knew but God. Each morning as I prepared breakfast and made school lunches for my kids, I prayed that I would not cry as I looked into their precious little faces. After they left the house each morning, I closed the door with great relief that I hadn't cried and that I now had time alone to grieve. I sat with my Bible, breakfast, and tears, and poured my heart out to God.

Initially, I felt the pangs of saying goodbye to my own life and dealing with the fear of death. Thankfully, many years prior, God's Spirit had confirmed in my spirit that I belonged to him, that Christ had cleansed me from my sin and my eternal salvation was secure. That security was a tremendous blessing. In addition, one morning during my most memorable devotion, I was reading a wonderful book on prayer and read a Scripture the author referenced that leapt off the page. The Scripture was Psalm 73:25: "Whom have I in heaven but you? And there is nothing on earth that I desire besides you. My flesh and my heart may fail, but God is the strength of my heart and my PORTION forever."

In the deepest part of my soul, I experienced a knowledge of God and a trust of him that I never imagined possible. All I could do was weep. The Holy Spirit was giving me full assurance that he was literally all I ever needed and that I did indeed have him and, therefore, I could not be any more blessed than I already was. With or without cancer, I was good. I could either be content having his life in me on earth, or I could be complete in him in heaven.

The decision was God's to make, and I told him that I trusted him completely to make the right decision. I asked him to heal me and allow me to remain a mother, wife, daughter, and friend, but if he wanted to take me home at age forty, I trusted him. This exchange and the gift of faith in him that he imparted has been the greatest miracle of my life. I remain forever changed by it.

My time in his presence continued as each day the reality hit me afresh that my children might lose their mother. The thought of leaving them without a mother and no longer being with them was too heart-wrenching to bear. I would read the Psalms until I could find my voice in their words. As I did, my tears would turn from tears of sadness to tears of utter joy. I could feel God's love for me so strongly that I couldn't contain it. His promise to always be with me overwhelmed my soul. He was filling my heart with the faith I so desperately needed to place my children in his care. I could fully trust my Shepherd and Lord with my family.

At times, it was as though I was in a bubble of sorts, hidden in the cleft of the rock, under his wings, in his shelter, and protected from fear and doubts that seemed always to be crouching at the door. Those hours spent crying out to him have been the most meaningful and fulfilling of all my life. It has now been nine years since my diagnosis, and I have continued to receive clear MRI scans every six months.

God's healing of my physical health in this dramatic way has been incredibly precious to me and to my family, and words cannot fully describe the richness of the time I spent in his presence experiencing His deep love for me. I tease people that I highly recommend a brain tumor! *I would not trade the trial* of going through brain cancer for the nearness to Christ I have experienced because of it.

A surrendered life to him brings more peace and joy than this world could ever give. He is our peace if we belong to him. It is so merciful of him to bring various tribulations into our lives. As Samuel Rutherford noted, "There is no sweeter fellowship with Christ than to bring our wounds and our sores to him." It is by his grace alone that I can say he is better than life itself. To God be the glory.

Charlotte's Story
Through the Valley

My cancer journey occurred when my husband and I were following God's call with the mission known as Overseas Crusade, now called One Challenge. We were living in the States, having returned from the Philippines and Singapore, representing the mission in various churches. My husband was on his way to New Jersey to speak, and he had dropped me off at my cousin's home in North Carolina. I discovered a lump in my breast, which totally surprised and shocked me. Looking back, I can see God's kindness to allow me to be in the home of my cousin, who is a nurse and whose husband is a physician. The fact that I wasn't alone and had their input and medical advice was a wonderful comfort and provision from God.

Fear was one of the main emotions I faced at the beginning. God was teaching me to rely on him in a deeper way. In March of 1988, I wrote out this prayer, "Father, I offer to you my fears of inadequacy and my inability to write and speak very well. I rely completely on you, my source and supply, to meet my need for security and significance.

As I proceeded forward in this unknown journey, the words of Elisabeth Elliot came back to me: "Do the next thing." I was also greatly encouraged by a book I read by Amy Carmichael: "Sometimes we wake feeling down and we feel like that all day long for no reason that we can discover-only that it is so. It is useless to try to feel different; trying does not touch feelings. It is useless to argue with oneself; feelings are like the mists that cover the mountains in misty weather. The mists pass: the mountains abide. Turn to your Father, tell him you know that he is with you whether you feel it or not... ."

The view of Jesus as the shepherd was a great comfort at this time as well. In Psalm 23, we read that the Lord walks with us through the valley. The important word in this sentence is "through." Notice it doesn't say, *into* the valley, or *over* the valley, or *down*, or even *up* the valley, but "*through* the valley." God doesn't take us out of the trial but is with us *through* it. The presence of the Shepherd is our peace and joy during the trial. The trial or time of suffering is a tunnel. Tunnels always have openings at both ends, the entrance and the exit. The Shepherd who brings us in will walk us through, and at the right time lead us out the exit. I wrote in my journal during this time, "To obey is the main thing. Success is God's job. My significance and worth are in Christ. The results are in his hand."

I saw God's faithfulness in many ways during the cancer journey, particularly through other people and the way he used their prayers. At another time, I prayed, "Lord, restore to me the joy of Thy salvation." Shortly after my prayer, a friend of mine called to say it was as if God pulled back the curtains of Heaven and showed her that he delights in my husband Keith and me. We are his joy, and he will use us greatly. Another friend said as she prayed, she believed God, upon bringing me through the cancer journey, would bring us into our fullest and most fruitful season of ministry yet.

After the cancer trial, we lived in Singapore for three years and then Hong Kong for another three years. We experienced a very fruitful time of God's blessing and the way he used us in these two countries.

It's been thirty-eight years since that incredible journey of walking with my Shepherd through the valley of cancer. He has been faithful.

Mary's Story
An Answer to Prayer to Hold on To

My story began in the shadow of a strong family history of breast cancer. My mother, aunt, and uncle were all diagnosed with breast cancer in their fifties. Then, when my older sister was diagnosed in her late forties, I also decided to be checked since I had pain in my left breast. At this time, I was homeschooling my three daughters, ages ten, seven, and five and caring for my young toddler. Anxiety and fear filled me from the start as I thought of the time it would take to get checked, and to get to all the appointments and tests, while at the same time caring for my young children.

This diagnosis in my early forties caused me great anxiety and fear. Fear of the unknown and trusting the Lord is often a great challenge for me. Although my husband was a great help and support during this time, I knew he struggled with the diagnosis as I did. I also felt overwhelmed with concern for my children and how to best help and care for them during this difficult time. God was teaching me to surrender my life more completely in trust to his care, especially for my children.

The decisions surrounding my breast cancer surgery were very complex and overwhelming, adding to my stress and fear. My sister had a prophylactic double mastectomy as well as an oophorectomy (removal of the ovaries) due to our family history and to reduce the chance of recurrent breast or possible ovarian cancer. However, my OB/GYN advised against oophorectomy because, among other benefits to keeping my ovaries, their removal would put me into menopause immediately, fifteen years before

I'd experience it naturally. Despite my doctor's advice, I decided to go ahead with the oophorectomy. Unfortunately, I let fear and others' decisions influence my decision-making process.

My first surgery consisted of a double mastectomy with reconstruction using a tram flap, that is, my own abdominal tissue, and small saline implant. It took about ten hours with two more lengthy surgeries and much time to heal. The thought of leaving my children for long periods of time, while making it through such long surgeries and recoveries, overwhelmed me. In fact, I was filled with shame because I viewed my fears and anxiety as a great weakness and displeasing to God. I believed my fear showed a lack of trust and belief in him. I was learning that God meets us where we are and grows our faith in the midst of our doubts and fears.

My dear friend's mother, Charlotte, whose story is just before this one, phoned and shared with me how God used a friend to encourage her that the Lord would "raise her up and that the best years of ministry alongside her husband were still ahead of her." After speaking to Charlotte, I prayed for something specific that God would give me that I could hold on to, something obvious that God would communicate to me to let me know everything would be ok. I kept this prayer between me and God and waited on him to answer.

I went to my pre-op appointment the day before the surgery and still had no answer from God. The drive home felt very lonely. Although I had great support from family and friends, no one but Jesus could take away my fears. When I got home, the friend who was watching my children shared that she had been praying for me during the previous weeks. She explained an image that God had put in her mind, "While you were on the operating table, Jesus was leaning over you. His face was right over you and his hair surrounded your face. He was touching your forehead and whispering in your ear like a loving father would that you are his and he will take care of you." She continued, saying, "The peace and tenderness I felt while praying was real, like nothing I've felt while praying before."

With this assurance and the specific way God met me where I needed him, I was full of peace. The image my friend shared, and her words were exactly what I needed to hear. *God had answered my prayer and given me what I needed to hold on to.*

Psalm 31:7 was very meaningful at this time and reflects what God did for me: "I will be glad and rejoice in your love, for you saw my affliction and knew the anguish of my soul." Just prior to the surgery, even my surgeon noticed my newfound joy and peace, and commented, "Well, you look happy!" I was able to laugh and smile, saying, "Jesus has me and I know I am going to be fine."

Jody's Story
Living with Stage Four

Mine might be the story no one really wants to read. Certainly not a story anyone wishes to experience. When I was diagnosed with breast cancer in 2011, it was stage one—in fact, *barely* stage one. After a double mastectomy, clear margins, clear lymph nodes, and ten years of tamoxifen treatment, my doctors gave me the "all clear!" For ten years, my doctors applauded me as The Poster Girl for Beating Breast Cancer. I did everything right, or so it seemed. For an entire decade, I marched forward believing cancer was in the rearview mirror for me and my family. But eleven years later, it found its way back.

On a random CT scan, for something entirely unrelated, spots were discovered in my spine. My doctors didn't believe it possible. One doctor sent me home and said not to worry, it just couldn't be cancer. But God prompted us to push further and after biopsying a lesion in my pelvis, I was delivered the crushing news that this was, indeed, the same breast cancer spread to my bones. I was brutally catapulted from barely stage one to stage four. I was catapulted from freedom to fear. I was catapulted from a peaceful life to a probable loss of life. *Metastatic, incurable* and *terminal* were now the words stamped on this Poster Girl's paperwork.

It was inconceivable. I had less than a 1% chance for recurrence. I was living life to the fullest. At fifty-three, I was still raising our five kids, active and athletic, involved and busy. I wasn't thinking about cancer's return. I wasn't thinking about cancer at all. I was chasing down the dreams of middle age and my next season of life. This news felt impossible.

Even today, two and half years from my stage-four diagnosis, I still wake some mornings thinking it must somehow be wrong. How does one go from poster girl to poor prognosis? I have cried out to God a million times. How? Why? Why me? What if? What now?

There was so much I didn't know about stage four. I never thought I'd need to know. We scrambled to understand what it all meant. The internet was a cruel teacher telling me I could expect to live three to five years after diagnosis. I read that. My husband read that. I am certain my kids Google-searched and read those same devastating words as well. How does a vibrant woman, volunteering everywhere and playing tennis each week with zero symptoms or pain all of a sudden find herself staring down three to five years of life ahead?

First and foremost, Google can be wrong. Those numbers and words are somewhat antiquated and, at the end of the day, only statistics. Google is not God. That's what I remember thinking early on. Google doesn't get to tell me how many days I have left; God does. "All the days ordained for me were written in your book before one of them came to be" (Psalm 139:16).

Yes, God is in complete charge of my days, but I had a part to play as well. "Teach us to number our days, that we might gain a heart of wisdom" (Psalm 90:12). I had a role to step into in this repulsive diagnosis. I was given news which got my attention. My days might be numbered—as all of our days are—but what was I going to do with that new information? How would God use it to give me a heart of wisdom? And isn't a heart of wisdom something so much greater than just chasing the paltry pleasures and wants of our world?

Is it possible that God has something more for me? Even in this pain. Even in this time left on earth. Yes. I am sure he does. It is important to include at this point that though those statistics are rough, women are living much longer with metastatic breast cancer. There is still no cure, but more and more treatments are surfacing all the time. My oncologist likes to tell me we are treating my stage-four cancer more as a chronic disease. But I assure you, chronic disease or not, it is not an easy one. The side effects are real. The constant scanning and testing and waiting for new results are absolutely exhausting.

Friends, unknowingly, ask, "Jody, when will your treatment end?" My answer is a hard one. "Never." I will always be in some kind of treatment. When scans show progression, we know the cancer has outsmarted my current treatment and it is time to change drugs. The goal is no longer to cure my cancer, but to extend my life. The sprint of finding a treatment to eradicate the disease has given way to a marathon of prolonging my days living with cancer. Unless Jesus supernaturally intervenes, my cancer will never go away. One doctor said of metastatic cancer that, "the horse has left the barn." The cancer cells hide mysteriously within my body. Our job now is to keep them sleepy and restrained.

In these past few years, I've learned a lot about stage-four breast cancer and I've also learned much about how Jesus meets us in the different stages of grief and suffering. It is too much for a short chapter at the end of this beautiful book, but, more than anything, I want to relay to readers that even when the news is as bad as it can be, all is not lost. Even when the results are not what we wished for, there is still hope. There is light and life even in the darkest places of this dreaded disease. Isaiah 45:3 says, "I will give you treasures hidden in the darkness—secret riches. I will do this so you may know that I am the Lord, the God of Israel, the one who calls you by name."

Treasures? Really? Strange as it seems, yes. For it is in the darkest places that we more deeply rely on Jesus. We find ourselves more desperate for his word, his ways, his worship. We are lost, so that we can be truly found in him. We are blind, so that we can see better his path. We are broken, so that we can be healed by his hand. We are crushed, so that we might better know his cross. It is the upside-down world of following Christ, as God's word repeatedly reminds us.

True treasure has little to do with the temporary fixes in which we find diversion, distraction, and dalliance. No, it is so much more. It is costly, but God's treasure has immeasurable value. It is worthy. Lasting. Eternal. Everything. Romans 8:17-18 encourages us, "then we are heirs—heirs of God and co-heirs with Christ, if indeed we share in his sufferings in order that we may also share in His glory."

Don't get me wrong. My flesh longs for the quick fixes and lighter luxuries of this world. For easy days. For comfort. For convenience. For the carefree. Those desires will never end this side of heaven, but my soul knows that it is in these dark places where treasure resides. I'd like to change that sometimes, but instead, I am learning to trust him more at all times.

Chapter 21
When Cancer Ends in Death

It is my hope that if you or your loved one is facing death caused by cancer, that this chapter will especially speak to you. Psalm 23:4 says, "Even though I walk through the valley of the shadow of death, I will fear no evil, for you are with me; your rod and your staff, they comfort me." (ESV) And Psalm 139:11, 12, "If I say, 'Surely the darkness will hide me and the light become night around me,' even the darkness will not be dark to you; the night will shine like the day, for darkness is as light to you."

God has already gone before us into our deepest and darkest valley. His presence and promises are sure and certain. Be assured that Jesus himself experienced this reality in the deepest way beyond any human's suffering when he died on the cross, bearing the weight of the sin of the world. His victory on the cross and over the grave by his resurrection, assures us of our own resurrection and that of our loved ones. God in his infinite love an mercy has given us this eternal hope and tangible comfort if our lives are united with Christ. This is why we can truthfully say that he is with us no matter what happens, and that our night can be as bright as the day.

The following story from my friend Amy underscores this truth and God's faithfulness.

Amy's Story
He is Truly Faithful

I tell a story that some may not want to hear. The cure for cancer didn't come in the way we wanted, longed for, or prayed for, but ultimately Tom was healed in heaven.

My husband Tom was diagnosed with stage 4 colon cancer at the age of twenty-nine. He was a healthy, strong Airborne Army Ranger and was my soulmate of four years and the father to our ten-month-old daughter when he was diagnosed. We were just beginning our life together when he was suddenly struck down with late-stage colon cancer. The doctors told us to get our affairs in order and that he only had three months to live. Gratefully, doctors are not the predictors or givers of life and God had other plans for Tom that included sixteen more years of life. But they were hard years. Years full of twenty-nine major surgeries, five different protocols of chemo, radiation, stem cell transplants, cancer vaccines, nutrition and supplement protocols, and every kind of cancer gismo that you can imagine. The treatments were endless. I am now thirteen years out from Tom's passing, and I still tremble remembering all the years of treatment and fighting he endured.

But God....

Cancer is an ugly enemy that doesn't fight fairly. If you are reading this book, you know that. But God made a way for us when it looked as if there was no way. He showed me my highest calling at that time was to love my husband through the hardest, most difficult part of his life. I learned to accept and embrace this calling as my life. We can waste life by wishing for the suffering to pass, wanting to get back to our normal life. Yet I knew this would mean missing all that God had for me. For He had grace that I never could have fathomed, and a life-giving presence that accompanied me in my darkest days.

There is so much I could say about this sixteen-year cancer journey and the thirteen years of widowhood and single parenting that have followed, but if I had to sum it up, I would tell you… **God is faithful**.

There were three life-changing lessons I learned during this time.

First, God demonstrates his faithfulness by preparing and equipping you for what He calls you to do.

1 Thessalonians 5:24 says, "Faithful is He who calls you, who also will do it." The year before Tom's diagnosis I read Jerry Bridges' book, <u>Transforming Grace</u>. I began to understand grace more fully. God does not treat us in the way we deserve but offers us forgiveness in Christ instead. Christ's sacrificial gift on the cross covers our sin and gives us his unmerited salvation. And God does not owe us anything. Just because I am a Christian does not mean my life will be easy. As Job 2:10 says "Shall we accept good from God and not trouble?" Tom's diagnosis helped me realize that I would have to stand before the throne of God, alone. It

challenged me to take accountability for my spiritual walk and not depend on my husband. In a lot of ways, my husband had become an idol, a type of savior in my life.

Second, we are able to better understand God's faithfulness by knowing God's character.

In order to trust God, we have to know him. We get to know him by spending time with him, reading about him, looking for him in and around us and studying his truths. When we know his character, it helps us trust him even when it doesn't make sense or is scary. His ways are not our ways, as Isaiah 55:8 describes, " 'For my thoughts are not your thoughts, neither are your ways my ways', declares the Lord."

It was not "my way" when in 2012, Tom passed away from cancer after his grueling sixteen-year battle at the age of forty-five. Our children were fourteen and sixteen. Life felt completely out of control. My greatest fear had come true. Tom didn't die as an Army Ranger in action. He died fighting another enemy, cancer. For me, fear now shifted to my kids getting cancer and I was determined to protect them with all that I had. Then, just three years later, my seventeen-year-old son was diagnosed with stage 3 cancer and was not given a good prognosis.

In these moments we need to remember God's character and trust Him for what is next, even when we don't understand. Martin Luther said, "I know not where He leads me, but well do I know my Guide."

Third, we remind ourselves of God's faithfulness by remembering what He has done.

In Joshua 4 we read that when God had faithfully brought the Israelites into the land he promised them, he had them gather twelve large rocks to form into a memorial which served for generations as a reminder of God's faithfulness.

God wants us to remember what he's done and testify to what he's accomplished. He wants us to hold on to his faithfulness when it's hard to face the present or the future. I don't know what the future holds. My son is still fighting cancer and doing daily treatments. I have no guarantee that just because I faced one heart-wrenching loss that I won't have to face another. Remembering God's abiding presence and his faithfulness to me in the past helps me hang on to that for the future. This is why in the scriptures God so often tells us, "Remember."

Tangible and visual reminders in my daily life help me remember God's faithfulness. I have a "jar of stones" that serve this purpose. I've collected twenty-nine years of stones, with a written testimony of God's care and work in my life, each a demonstration of his grace and character being played out in my heart, and each a reminder when fears or doubts arise.

Several of these read:
"God provided for medical bills."
"He makes all things new."
"He gave dear widow friends."
"God provided a new job."
"The gift of togetherness on a family vacation."
"God is my Redeemer."
"A dog to adopt, named Mercy, to remind us of God's mercy."
"Clarity of cancer treatment for Nate."
"Wonderful spouses for both my children."
"Courage for me to go on a date."

So, what will you tell your children of how God has been faithful to you? 1 Peter 3:14 says, "Do not fear...do not be frightened. But in your hearts revere Christ as Lord. Always be prepared to give an answer to everyone who asks you to give the reason for the hope you have." For this reason, I'm sharing my testimony with you now.

After eight years of being a widow and single mother, God demonstrated his faithfulness to me yet again in recent years by bringing my husband into my life. This is another testimony of God's grace. He has allowed me to love again and share the burden of life with someone. I want to encourage you to look for ways that God is equipping you. Spend time with God and know his character so you can learn to trust him more. Remember what he has done, testify to it and hold on to him, for he is truly faithful!

Chapter 22
Practical Tips

Before closing, I'd like to pass on a few practical tips and things I'm glad I did to help during my cancer journey.

"I'm glad I sent out email/text updates."
The night before each chemo session and surgery, I sent out a brief email or text message to friends asking for prayer. Not only did this raise up a lot of prayer, but it lifted my spirits before surgery or chemo to read all the encouraging messages. The replies let me know I was not alone. I had a community of support, and many were before the throne of God interceding on my behalf.

"I'm glad I said yes to meals."
Most of us are afraid to impose or ask for help, feeling it will cause a lot of work and trouble for others. But when I had a few friends and neighbors ask if they could bring meals, I knew this would meet a big need. When we say *yes* to others, we are building community and giving others the chance to give, serve, and love. Independence leads to isolation. Humility and openness to others lead to life-giving community and relationships. Also, as we open our lives to others, we will likely have the opportunity to serve them at some point in the future.

"I'm glad I was honest with my kids' questions."
Our teens had tough questions that needed honest answers: "Mom, are you going to die?" "Will your hair fall out?" "Will you be in bed a lot?" I was thankful for their questions because they were on my mind too. Thinking of how to communicate helpful and honest answers caused me to reflect on each one and enabled us all to face reality with candor and courage.

My answers sounded something like this:

"Yes, death comes for all of us, we just don't know when. Any of us could be in an accident tomorrow. If I die soon, I am confident that God will work this out and provide for you. He will fill in the gaps and be with you. The main thing is that we trust him and keep an open heart of faith and look to him."

"Yes, with chemo, my hair will fall out. I know I will feel really bad about that since I love my hair." (This was before I knew about cold caps, which I'll mention later.) "I will have to look for some fancy hats and scarfs. I'm glad real beauty is what's inside and that this is temporary. I'm going to pray that God gives me perspective to focus on that."

"Chemo may be rough, and there may be certain days where I won't be able to do much. I am sure we will all pitch in together and figure out what to do. God will give us wisdom to know how best to get things done. With all the meals coming in from the neighbors, at least we won't starve to death!" Adding humor at the right time helped us put the problem into perspective. We saw our kids, together with us, learning to trust God with these uncertainties, which pushed us further in our spiritual growth. If you have kids at home, you know truthful and honest answers said in theage-appropriate way will open the door for God to do his work. Side-stepping their questions or giving them pat answers don't help them learn to grapple with the hard questions of trusting God.

"I'm glad I thought about the location and timing for my treatments and appointments."
The many appointments to the infusion center, the doctors' visits, and daily excursions to radiation mean a lot of time spent in the car as well as time away from your normal routine. I made sure to look for doctors and places for treatment that were nearby and at times that fit into my schedule. Having the appointments as early as possible in the morning also meant they were most likely running on schedule with decreased wait times.

I'm glad I tried a cold cap."
A cold cap is used to prevent hair loss during chemo. Many hospitals or infusion centers have a contractual agreement with one of the cold cap companies to provide this for their patients. It worked very well for me, and I kept most of my hair. Cold caps are expensive, and insurance rarely pays for them, but keeping my hair was a pleasant surprise, and helped me emotionally through the chemo treatments and months afterwards.

A few important factors helped with the success of the cold cap:

First, make sure you follow all the directions. In addition, make sure your scalp is very wet when you put on the cap. I spent time at the infusion center dousing my hair in the sink in the bathroom with water till my scalp was soaking. I brought several hand towels to wipe up all the water on the bathroom floor and sink—and a couple to keep my back from getting soaked.

Second, use conditioner, leave it in, and brush it as flat as possible like the directions tell you, then put on the cap.

Third, make sure it is very snug all over, then secure it with the ties or bungees. It's better to go with a smaller size to make sure it is snug. The part on the crown often pops up a little, but a smaller size should prevent this. Remember, too, that it must be very tightly tied down and will feel uncomfortable at first.

Fourth, remember, the cap is designed to be cold—just above freezing to prevent blood circulation of the chemo from reaching the hair follicle cells, thus preventing them from dying and releasing the hair. When the cold cap machine is turned on, expect several minutes of a cold rush, but stick with it and try to read or do something else to distract yourself until you get used to it.

Fifth, have your electric heating blanket on hand. It provides a whole new definition of comfort and warmth during this time!

Closing

As I write this, a year has passed since I crossed the finish line of my cancer journey. The chemo, the radiation, the surgeries-they are now chapters behind me. What remains are the routine scans every six months and a few slowly fading scars. But even as those physical reminders soften, I've learned not to let the fresh joy and clarity I've received fade with them. Through it all, God breathed a new gratitude into my heart—a quiet but steady joy at the beauty of ordinary days, and a sharpened vision of eternal perspective. When I begin to forget these precious gifts from God, I pause and ask him for help. Through the scripture, his Holy Spirit, prayer, fellowship with other believers, and serving him, God is always faithful to pour out his grace and strength to walk in these realities again.

It is my earnest desire that this book has encouraged and helped you along your journey. If this is the case, or if you have any questions, I'd love to hear from you. Please email me through my blogspot page by going to:

https://valeriehuff.blogspot.com

Citations

1. Strong's Exhaustive Concordance Greek and Hebrew. 979, bios. www.biblehub.com. May 2024
2. Ibid., 5590, psuche.
3. Ibid., 2222, zoe.
4. C.S. Lewis, *Mere Christianity* (Harper One, 1952) p.159.
5. Strong's Exhaustive Concordance Greek and Hebrew. 4053, perissos. www.biblehub.com.
6. W. Phillip Keller, *A Shepherd's Look at Psalm 23* (Zondervan, 1970) p.26.
7. Elisabeth Elliot, *A Path Through Suffering* (Tyndale House Publishers, 2003) p.98.
8. Elisabeth Elliot, *Shadow of the Almighty: The Life and Testimony of Jim Elliot* (Harcourt, Brace and Company, 1958) p.173.
9. Elisabeth Elliot, *Keep a Quiet Heart* (Tyndale House Publishers, 1995) p.82.
10. The History of 'Disease'. Wordplay. WWW.Merriam-Webster.com. May 2024
11. Brother Lawrence, *The Practice the Presence of God* (Whitaker House, 1982) 2nd Letter, p.16, 17.
12. Tony Reinke, *12 Ways Your Phone is Changing You* (Crossway, 2017) p.44, 45.
13. C.S. Lewis, *Mere Christianity* (Harper One, 1952) p.3-32.
14. Francis A. Schaeffer, *How Should We Then Live? The Rise and Decline of Western Thought and Culture* (Fleming H. Revell, 1976) p.20.
15. C.S. Lewis, *The Problem of Pain* (Geoffrey Bles, 1940) Chapter: Divine Goodness.
16. Joni Eareckson Tada, *A Place of healing: Wrestling with the Mysteries of Suffering, Pain, and God's Sovereignty* (David C. Cook, 2010) p.49.

17. G.K. Chesterton, Orthodoxy, The Ethics of Eifland Essay (DLB Press, 2023, originally by Chatto & Windus, 1917).
18. Strong's Exhaustive Concordance Greek and Hebrew. 4239, prauteti, www.biblehub.com.
19. C.S. Lewis, *The Weight of Glory and Other Addresses* (Macmillan, 1949) p.1-3.
20. Timothy Keller, *Walking with God Through Pain and Suffering* (Penguin Random House, 2016) p.151.

Made in the USA
Coppell, TX
13 February 2026

72015376R10075